Advance Pra...
Obese from the Heart

"*Obese from the Heart* made me cry, and made me laugh. It touches upon so many things we as humans live with, or without. Sara Stein has an ability to speak to everyone, young and old, rich and poor, any race, religion, or gender."

> ~ Pamela Heller, Photographer
> http://PamelaHeller.com

"This book is almost lyrical, almost like a wonderful song. It has a rhythm to it that is entirely appropriate and unchanging throughout. Severely wonderful! "

> ~ Louise Hoffman, RN
> Bariatric Case Manager
> Kaiser Permanente

"I wasn't going to read this until I had a bit more time, but I couldn't help glancing at it....and I didn't stop until it was finished. *Obese from the Heart* is marvelous. Sara Stein writes with unequaled candor, wry humor and vivid story-telling. I congratulate you from the bottom of my heart."

> ~ Philippa Kennealy MD MPH CPCC PCC
> www.entrepreneurialMD.com

Obese from the Heart

A Fat Psychiatrist Discloses

Sara L. Stein, M.D.

Quantum Psych INK, LLC

Sara L. Stein, M.D.
c/o Quantum Psych INK, LLC
P.O. Box 241250
Cleveland, OH 44124
Phone / FAX (888) 898-8571
Email: info@obesefromtheheart.com
www.obesefromtheheart.com

ISBN - 10: 0982524811 (print)
ISBN - 13: 9780982524817 (print)

Library of Congress Control Number: 2009908302

Limits of Liability and Disclaimer of Warranty

The author and publisher shall not be liable for your misuse of this material. This book is strictly for informational and educational purposes.

Warning – Disclaimer

The purpose of this book is to educate and entertain. The author and/or publisher do not guarantee that anyone following these techniques, suggestions, tips, ideas, or strategies will become successful. The author and/or publisher shall have neither liability nor responsibility to anyone with respect to any loss or damage or injury caused, or alleged to be caused, directly or indirectly by the information contained in this book and/or related programs.

This book and/or website are not a substitution for appropriate psychological and medical treatment. Please consult with qualified medical personnel regarding the personal safety of using information found in this book and/or related programs. If you or someone you know is at risk of harming themselves or others, or unable to care for themselves, please seek emergency treatment or call 911.

The purchase and/or perusal of this book do not engage the purchaser/buyer in a physician-patient relationship with the author or her representatives. All forms of communication in response to this publication are not considered medical record and are therefore not subject to HIPPA regulation or privacy.

About The Author

Sara L. Stein, M.D., is a psychiatrist, author, speaker, and teacher. Her witnessing reflects the soul within both patient and doctor. These are not the stories of individuals, but the collective wisdom of working with thousands of people of all ages and all walks-of-life who struggle with their lives. Some struggle with addictions, some with circumstances, some with biology, but all with a need for greater healing than our currently overtaxed medical system can offer.

Dedication

This book is dedicated to the women and men who surround me in life and in spirit. For my mother, Marjorie, and her mother, Rose, and my nanny Genell, whose powerful female energies guide me through my every intention. To my dearest husband, Don, who lives hearing the rhythms of the universe. To my beloved family alive and in spirit; my father, Robert, my grandparents, sisters, aunts, uncles, nieces and nephews, who provide me an unending well of warmth and support and who challenge me to be my best. To my many friends, present, past and future, who give me a piece of their hearts and sustain me through hard times. To my teachers, coaches and mentors who open their minds and pour out their wisdom so I can find a better way. To my colleagues and staff who rise to every opportunity and are tireless in their caring.

To my beloved Newfoundlands who lie at my feet when I work and remind me when it's time to play.

But most of all, this is dedicated to the thousands of patients over the years, who feed my hunger for the magnificence of the human spirit and leave me feeling fuller and fuller everyday.

I do not know everything there is to teach, but I will teach you everything I know.

Acknowledgements

They don't teach book writing or storytelling in medical school. For their incredible expertise and assistance along this long and winding road, I'd like to thank my:

Book Cover Artist and Web Designer:
Lisa McLymont, www.veryidealdesign.com

Cover Design and Interior Layout:
Susan Daffron, www.logicalexpressions.com

Editor:
Laura Cross, www.ScenarioWritingStudio.com

Photographer:
Pamela Heller, http://PamelaHeller.com

Web Designer:
Nicholas Byfleet, www.nicholasbyfleet.com

Mentor and Coach
Philippa Kennealy M.D., M.P.H.
www.entrepreneurialMD.com

Book Coaches
Susan Daffron, www.logicalexpressions.com
Donna Kozik, www.mybigbusinesscard.com

Readers
Linda DeBalzo, R.N., C.N.S.,
Rachel Glass, M.Ed.

Contents

About The Author i

Dedication ii

Acknowledgements iii

Introduction 1

Section One 3

Chapter 1: The Curse Of Obesity 5

Chapter 2: Evolution Of An Addiction: When I Grow
Up I Want To Be A Chocolate Chip Cookie 9

Chapter 3: It Runs In My Family – I Was Doomed
Before I Was Even Born 15

Chapter 4: Stress – Running on Empty 21

Chapter 5: Depression – Vital Exhaustion 27

Chapter 6: Anxiety – I Can't Make It Stop 35

Chapter 7: Anger – Feeding the Fire Inside and Out 43

Chapter 8: The Black Hole of Trauma 49

Chapter 9: On Dying, Grief And Eating: The Abyss
of Emptiness 53

Section Two 59

Chapter 10: Counterfeit Energy: Can Food Actually
Keep Your Engine Running? 61

Chapter 11: The Last Chance Surgeries 65

Chapter 12: Somewhere Over The Rainbow:
Disconnected From Your Inner Self 69

Section Three 75

Chapter 13: Life Begins Tomorrow, I'll Start When
I'm Thin 77

Chapter 14: Sex And Love: They Fixed Me Up With
The Fat Kid 81

Chapter 15: Black Is My Favorite Color: The
Price Tag of Shame..87

Section Four **91**

Chapter 16: If You Know So Much, Why Are You
Still Fat?...93

Chapter 17: I'm Only Allowed Ten Grapes:
Is the Medical Community Helping or Hurting?......................97

Chapter 18: Where Do I Begin?..103

Chapter 19: The Last Unanswered Prejudice:
You Are Not Alone 109

Section Five **115**

Chapter 20: This Is What I Maybe Know For Sure 117

Resources 119

Introduction

Who is this book for?

Maybe it's easier to tell you whom it's NOT for.

If you are looking for a good diet, consider these suggestions:

If you have a few pounds to lose, try a balanced diet with meal plans or suggestions that suit your lifestyle - join a gym, go for a walk, stop drinking soda, drink tea, find a diet buddy or online support group, practice relaxation.

If you have a significant amount of weight to lose, go to your doctor, a nutritionist and start moving, even a little. Learn how to lose weight the healthy way, and try it. Make sure you do not have a medical condition that is causing the extra weight.

The rest of you, read on.

Read on if you are morbidly obese by medical standards and you have not successfully managed your weight.

Read on if you feel hopeless, helpless and defeated by your weight and your attempts to lose it.

Read on if your appearance does not reflect the way you feel inside.

Read on if others have reacted to your appearance before you even said one word to them.

Read on if you feel alone because of your weight or if your weight is a response to feeling alone.

Read on if the pounds you gain reflect the pain and emptiness you feel in life.

Read on if you have put your life on hold because of your weight or you have resigned yourself to living a better life in some other year or in some other universe.

Read on if you believe you are going to die because of your weight and you have not been able to change your ways.

Read on if you feel that there is an inner you clamoring to emerge; the you that accurately reflects your soul, the you that looks the way you feel.

This book is as much my story as your story. They are not different. We may have been born in different cities or countries; we may eat different foods or work in different vocations. We may worship with different languages and customs. We may be different ages and different sizes.

Underneath our exteriors, we are all the same. We love, we hate, we celebrate, we grieve. We play, we learn, we create. We have relationships that sustain us throughout our physical lives – relationships with people, with ourselves, with food, with our spiritual selves.

In the end, all we have are our relationships.

If I believe that my body serves to keep me separate from you, then I can never be connected to you, even in intimacy. We are connected by our emotions, by our energy, not by our bodies. Anyone who has ever felt another person's joy or suffering, whether in person or in the media, feels that connection. Why else would we weep over illnesses, or wars, or disasters, or crimes that affect those we have never met, in places we have never been?

We are all connected. My health reflects your energy. My love is an expression of your loyalty. My blessing is the song of your heart. And so it goes. When you are tired, I am in pain. When you are alone, I weep. When I am isolated from the flow of the universe, I cannot fill up, no matter how much I eat.

Section One

The Curse Of Obesity

When I Grow Up I Want To Be A Chocolate Chip Cookie

It Runs In My Family –

I Was Doomed Before I Was Even Born

Stress – Running On Empty

Depression – Vital Exhaustion

Anxiety – I Can't Make It Stop

Anger – Feeding The Fire Inside And Out

The Black Hole Of Trauma

On Dying, Grief And Eating: The Abyss of Emptiness

Chapter

1

The Curse Of Obesity

"And I saw Sisyphus at his endless task, raising his prodigious stone with both his hands.

With hands and feet he tried to roll it up to the top of the hill, but always, just before he could roll it over on to the other side, its weight would be too much for him, and the pitiless stone would come thundering down again on to the plain. Then he would begin trying to push it uphill again, and the sweat ran off him, and the steam rose after him."

— *The Odyssey",*
translated by Samuel Butler

The first thing you notice when you come into my office is me. All of me. At times, there has been more of me; other times less, but you always absorbed the same impression. The psychiatrist is fat. I am the psychiatrist. My body is fat. At times in my life, I tried to pretend it was not the truth; other times I chose to simply ignore it. I would do my utmost to disregard the *"surprise in your eyes when you saw my size"*. A nursery rhyme of consternation on your part, sometimes disdain.

For a while my size was my best tool, my humanness on display for all to see, my imperfection, my failure, my mistakes. You tell me about your inability to quit some habit. "Yes", I say, motioning toward my body, "I understand." I tell you right then-and-there, "Do I look like I know all the answers?" I am not a doctor who dictates how you should live, I told myself. But really it was just an excuse for my inability to manage my own struggle with weight. I wanted to tell you how to live. I just had to learn how myself.

What an extraordinary shock that must have been for you. If the doctor doesn't have the answer, then who does? How can the doctor help me if she cannot even help herself? I wondered the same thing. I accepted the responsibility and ethical commitment as a healer, and *yet, I could not help myself even when it was the only right thing to do.*

In the chubby women's section of the store, the surprise works the other way – my size is a presumption of failure in life. "You're a doctor?" the same-size sales clerks would ask incredulously, as they rang up my size 26 pants. I heard their unspoken words "How can that be? Look at you!! You're fat!" And their implied thoughts, "There's hope for me, yet. If she can do it, I can, too." We are our own, and each other's, worst enemies.

I tried. I dieted. I exercised. I led an active normal life -the fat girl swimming, skiing, and dancing. I lost weight. I gained weight. I quit dieting. I quit exercising. I went to diet camp. I went to psychiatrists. I took medication. I stopped medication. I craved and withstood. I craved and indulged. I denied my size. I accepted my size. I read a thousand books and took a hundred different supplements. My body only got bigger and sicker; my spirit withered. I developed diabetes, edema, hypothyroid, psoriasis, liver problems, sleep apnea, sinus congestion, chronic pain, depression, brain fog and attention deficit. Every step hurt. I drove around looking for parking spaces close to the entrance, praying for working elevators and short hallways. I snored like a freight train and was always exhausted.

I had a wonderful doctor who tolerated my resistance and offered me help every time I saw him. When I went.

Like Sisyphus, I pushed the rock uphill, but it always came tumbling back down upon me.

It culminated one night when I thought I had a small stroke. One night, I felt a little pop deep inside my brain. No sensation, no sound, just a pop. It awoke me suddenly and painlessly. I knew. The next day one hand didn't grasp quite as strongly as the other. One eyelid seemed weaker. And with all of the powers of faith and denial inside me, I made two decisions:

1. I decided I did not want to die.
2. I decided I did not want to go to the doctor yet. I knew what I had to do. There was nothing wrong with my medication. The problem was me. I wasn't taking it. I wasn't doing what I needed to do.

In my heart, I knew that I could recover. I just did not know how. At the core of my very being, I believe that our bodies are healing machines. My machine was in serious disrepair, and I needed to get it running again. Or I would die from my weight.

This was my test of faith.

I knew the illness inside of me was my own creation. The sum of years and years of harming myself with my lifestyle. This purposeful not listening to my body, not caring, intending to do harm was not simply my internal organs aging and ailing. I knew what was inside of me was a reflection of something larger than physical. I just didn't know what it was.

I didn't know how to change what I was doing. Up to this point, my life experience seemed to be a series of what had not worked. This is the story of how I arrived in this tragic place and how I regained my life, and my spirit and my health. Inch by inch, ounce by ounce, pound by pound, one moment at a time.

My life is a weave of mind and body and spirit.

I had to learn how to love.

I had to learn how to give and forgive.

I had to learn how to thank.

I had to learn what to eat so I was satisfied, learn how to move my body in a way that was energizing, and learn how to rest so that I am replenished.

There is no right way to become healthy and whole. There is no one way to live. But if you have an ounce of wish left inside you, I invite you to come along with me for the rest of this journey.

Chapter

2

Evolution Of An Addiction: When I Grow Up I Want To Be A Chocolate Chip Cookie

When I was 3 years old, I spent every Saturday afternoon with my grandmother. Those few hours defined the entire week. Any activity we chose was fine; our joy was in being together, no matter what we did for fun. On nice days we would take a walk up to the shopping strip. We talked and sang. She would tell me stories about the "olden" days. I would look at shiny makeup cases in the Five and Dime or smell pungent shoe polish in Sam's Shoe Repair. We would stroll past the bowling alley and listen to the satisfying crack of falling pins and people laughing.

My only addiction until that point was those afternoons.

This particular day, the sun was shining. It was finally spring. For the first time in months, I didn't have a coat on. I felt free, and light and full of life. We stopped into the bakery, where lively talking women and a few men were filling their brown paper bags with newspapers and rye breads. The scent of pumpernickel and warm sugar intoxicated me. From behind the counter, a lady with a heavy accent handed me a giant, freshly baked chocolate chip cookie in a crinkly tissue paper.

It was the perfect storm.

One bite of that cookie, a sublimely baked combination of love and sweetness and sun and fun and fascination and conversation, one bite of that cookie and my little brain exploded in ecstasy. It was more feel good serotonin, dopamine and oxytocin in my brain than I had ever experienced in my life. Even in a good life.

I had just become addicted. That's all it took. I wasn't weak or ill intended. I was just a little girl in love with her grandmother who ate a cookie on a sunny day.

A lady stopped to greet my grandmother, and admire me.

"What do you want to be when you grow up, Sara?" she asked.

"A chocolate chip cookie", I responded, and continued munching without interruption.

The two grandmothers laughed heartily at my three-year old sense of humor.

Only I was serious. For months, maybe even years afterwards, I secretly imagined myself growing up and turning into a bakery chocolate chip cookie. It was a deeply satisfying fantasy.

I wasn't a fat three-year old. I was an ADDICTED three-year old. My little brain had just exploded a brain chemistry reward bomb in response to grandmotherly love and bakery cookies. I now had a new life's goal. The pursuit of dopamine, serotonin, oxytocin and norepinephrine, nature's way of making you feel like you won the lottery. And I knew where to find it. At the bakery. With my grandmother. On a sunny Saturday. In the chocolate chip cookies. Maybe just in the chocolate chips.

Getting the second chemical bomb wasn't that easy, I discovered. The feeling wasn't as intense the next week. No matter how hard I tried, no matter how many cookies I finagled out of my poor grandmother (and aunt, and mother and other grandmother and friends' mothers), no matter how often I hit pay dirt, the feeling wasn't the same.

The only difference between the food addict and the alcoholic or cocaine addict or gambler or the shopaholic or the sex addict is the drug of choice: Food.

Chocolate, and fries, and pizzas and chips can give you an incredible high and leave you wanting more, followed by a desperate crash that leaves you feeling depressed, anxious, and exhausted .

Food addiction is unique among addictions in four ways:

Food is unavoidable.

Food is essential for life.

Food is socially acceptable, everywhere.

Food can actually elevate your status if it's good!

It gets worse though…food is the only addicting substance where abstinence is both impossible and socially UNACCEPTABLE everywhere. It's not just "don't drink in a bar", it's everyone noticing that you are not eating. Especially the cook.

So begins the brutal cycle of trying to control your addiction while still using. DIEting…..

Quickly I learned the first lesson of addiction. One cookie wasn't enough. I kept trying to get that feeling again, but when I ate another cookie a week later my eager brain wasn't acting so eager. It no longer poured out the torrent of feel-good chemicals that had made me so euphoric only seven days earlier. Actually, the feel-good chemicals kind of dribbled out as feeling not-too-bad chemicals. At first they dribbled out one bite at a time, then it took an entire cookie, then two, then a row, then a box. As the weeks and months went by, the chemical stream dried up. You get the idea. It was taking more and more cookies to get the same feel-good in my brain. Meanwhile, my little body was getting fatter and fatter.

Every candy bar in every store spoke my name. My goal was to clean the shelves, like cleaning my plate. The only way I could calm myself was by realizing that they would still be there tomorrow. Lesson number two of addiction. Must have it. Need it. Gotta get some. NOW. Anxiety about getting the substance.

Lesson number three was the story of my life from that moment on. The big negative consequence of addiction? Nature never leaves anything the same; the universe is constantly expanding outward. So was my waist.

Even though I didn't want to be fat, even though I wished I was thin, even though I liked physical activity, even though I wanted to be normal, even though I was unhappy about gaining weight…I wanted that cookie chemistry feeling more. No matter how miserable I became.

I don't know if it is comforting or disturbing to realize that my food addiction did not start because of an event, or a character flaw or a genetic consequence. My food addiction began because I had a really big brain response to a really average occurrence.

Maybe it would have been better if I started overeating because of some horrible event or an awful feeling about myself. I could have run to the mental health professionals for treatment and closure.

THE FOURTH LAW OF ADDICTION

There is a FOURTH law of addiction that most addicts soon come to realize. Besides cravings, and withdrawal, and tolerance, and no longer caring about consequences, there is the LAW OF DEPRESSION. Cocaine addicts understand this law well, they get high then they crash. They sleep for a day or two and feel better. With each crash they become more depressed and with each recovery they feel less improved.

You know this one, too, you just never put it together as a side effect of the FOOD; most of us think it's a response to guilty pleasures. The day after a binge, when you are weepy or sad or even suicidally depressed, it's not entirely because you went off a diet or gained a pound. Your brain and body are having a physical response to all that food.

Your body is exhausted, your brain is spinning and depleted, your cells and organs have overworked themselves attempting to provide enough insulin for all that sugar, and to get rid of all the toxins in all that food. Your body's vitamins and minerals are depleted and are not restored by the junk you have eaten.

You feel like dying. Not like you are dying. Like you would rather be dead. Heavy, and sad, and worthless and hopeless.

There actually might be a little good news here. Some of the depression might be coming from what you ate. Which makes it very treatable.

But how do you provide treatment for an essential, beautiful moment of life? How do you train your brain NOT TO BE SO HAPPY? And not to want that happiness again and again?

You can't.

And you shouldn't try to deny yourself joy.

Your brain is a joy machine. It has all the ability to bliss-you-out for hours naturally.

What I had to learn was: what ELSE besides food would provide that explosion of joy. And what else would make it last and heal my body in the process?

Your body releases dopamine in response to pleasurable activities, including food, sex, sleep, exercise, laughing, singing, painting, and gardening.

Your body releases acetylcholine and GABA for relaxation in response to quieting your mind through meditation, prayer, yoga, and petting your animal.

Anytime and anywhere you want, you can fill your day with moments that fuel your brain at no extra cost to your wallet and no expense to your body.

The more you substitute these activities for food, the less you will eat.

In the following chapters, I will talk about emotions, and events and people that energize our eating, drain our will, and sabotage our efforts.

For today, simply identify one activity in your life that has the potential to bring you joy, other than food. Almost everyone, even the most depressed and anxious people can identify something or someone they love that makes them feel good for a moment. That is where we start.

Chapter 3

It Runs In My Family – I Was Doomed Before I Was Even Born

"There are very few human beings who receive the truth,complete and staggering, by instant illumination.

Most of them acquire it fragment by fragment, on a small scale, by successive developments, cellularly, like a laborious mosaic."

— *Anais Nin*

I see pictures of my paternal grandmother. She is 40ish and very obese. Easily 150 pounds overweight. My dad, the youngest of six, is a round little boy of four or five years old, and comes up to her waist. The family resemblance is both clear and implied. A blend of kitchen goodness and familial fat. Her house was filled with the smell of food made from scratch, the kind of food that worked both the muscles in her arms and the love in her heart. Hours of chop and grind and slice and stir and taste. She had the biggest soupspoons for eating I have ever seen. They might have been serving spoons, but probably they reflected how hard my bricklaying grandfather worked everyday. Each spoonful held a quarter-cup of chicken broth and noodles and vegetables. You could taste the quantity of love for her family in every bowl.

But now I look at that picture and see a woman who left her family with a young husband and new baby and moved half a world away. In a time when there was no communication, no phone, no Internet, no postal service that would ensure mail delivery across three continents. In a time when staying meant danger, even death. In a time when leaving meant never seeing your family again. Ever. In a time when she would raise her daughters without her grandmother and mother and aunts to guide her. In a time when her sons would not have the wisdom that grandfathers give to young boys.

How do you walk away from the people you love into a world of the unknown, knowing that you will never see them again? That you may never hear from them again? That you won't see your mother or father hold their grandchildren, or celebrate holidays or family happiness? You do that to give your children a better life, but what taste do you have deep in your soul from that level of loss? When did people who emigrated get news of their mothers and fathers dying? How long did it take news to get from rural Tsarist Russia to Ohio in the early 1900's? Now that I am grown and older, I understand the cavernous empty feeling of loneliness she must have had in her heart. There was no amount of food that would ever fill that void. Not even 100 extra pounds worth.

This isn't a story of genetics. This is a story of separation and loss. And the bottomless hole it leaves inside of you.

Is it possible that the genetics of food addiction are related more to our family stories than to our chromosomes?

The genetics of obesity are not about physical body; they are the genetics of inherited emotion, tied intimately to the stories of our families and passed along in our cultures, mouthful-by-mouthful.

I look at my grandmothers (both overweight) and consider the legacy of their stories:

IT IS PROBABLY NOT GENETIC – THEREFORE, IT'S NOT HOPELESS

Is that good news or bad news to you?

We are a generation of medical practitioners and patients raised on "genetic determinism". "I have high cholesterol because it's in my genes. Being big runs in my family. All of my father's side has depression – there's no escaping it."

And while there is a great deal of truth to the genetics of our bodies and our minds, genes alone DO NOT explain why we are obese or unhealthy.

Let's take cancer as an example. Science has been able to isolate genes that cause breast and ovarian cancer. Blood tests can identify individuals that have those genes.

BUT NOT ALL OF THE WOMEN WITH BREAST-OVARIAN CANCER GENES GET CANCER!!!!

So much for genetic determinism. It's not a sure thing. It's more like genetic predisposition…….

I treat people all the time who have slightly elevated cholesterols and think they have genetic high cholesterol. "No, you probably don't", I tell them. This lab value is about what you eat, how you move, and how your body processes the food. This is how much stress you're under and how hard it is for you to relax. This is genetics of culture and lifestyle, not simply DNA.

My father's mother left her family at the age of 18, never to see them again. Some of her family died in the village persecutions of Russia. Others died in Holocaust. Her first child died. Years later when my father's cousin painted our house, he told stories of the Warsaw Ghetto and the concentration camps to my toddler niece in the playpen.

My mother's mother was raised in an orphanage where her 5 year-old little brother died of tuberculosis. She cared for her invalid mother who suffered a stroke and died in her 40's, while my grandmother was still a very young woman.

My grandparents lost their house in the Great Depression.

I grew up listening to my grandmother tell the story of how my uncle was lost at sea during World War II when his destroyer was torpedoed and sunk in the South Pacific. And how, two weeks later, the postman ran down the street waving a telegram and shouting, "He's alive! Marvin's alive!" 50 years later, she still wept when she told the story.

I learned stories of my people's slavery and generations of oppression and murder year after year.

While we told the stories, we ate.

While we grieved, we ate.

While we celebrated, we remembered the dead and we ate.

We lived with a responsibility to remember those we lost and to heal the world from evil, and we ate.

It was a personal and a cultural statement. We stand on the shoulders of generations of suffering. In their honor and in their memory, this food sustains us and we cherish and bless this celebration.

It was an emotion of pain that passed through generations. In song, and stories, and expressions, in hands that shook imperceptibly as the food was ladled out. Tears that never spilled over when birthday candles were blown out. Never again. They must never be forgotten.

This is the genetics of obesity in my family, the way I felt it.

Every culture, every race, every religion, every nationality, every town, every family, every person has pain in their history. We are storytellers and teachers by nature. We know what is important and what must be remembered. However, remembering their stories and suffering their pain are not the same.

Parents do not wish for their children to suffer more than they did.

We pass along the defining moments of our lives generation to generation. When all that remains is pain and helplessness, the listener begins to suffer. It becomes a form of secondary trauma. The generationally obese person turns to food for relief and comfort.

You do not have to be obese because those before you were obese. Whether or not you have to suffer their memories is not my decision to make. If you are carrying around pounds of intergenerational suffering and memory, tell the story of your family or your culture, and then leave it go. The next generation will thank you for embracing health rather than suffering.

Chapter

4

Stress – Running on Empty

"Nobody on his deathbed ever said,'I wish I had spent more time at work.' "

— *unknown*

"I'm late, I'm late for a very important date

No time to say, "Hello", "Goodbye"

I'm late, I'm late, I'm late, I'm late."

— *Sammy Fain and Bob Hilliard (from the Walt Disney film,"Alice In Wonderland")*

Stress is society's greatest modern affliction. We have completely lost control of our workdays. A workday used to be dawn to dusk. It used to be from the time you arrived at your workplace until you went home. It used to be 5 days a week. Not anymore. We work constantly, 24 hours a day, 7 days a week. We work at our jobs, in our homes, at school, in traffic, at the grocery store. We work shopping on the Internet.

When we are resting, we are working: making lists, setting goals, reviewing today, and planning for tomorrow. We are not resting.

We continually increase our workload because work is addicting. We physically experience an increase in adrenalin, and energy and focus that expands our productivity. It's a rewarding feeling to do a good job at something.

We add more work so we can feel even better. We start multi-tasking: the dishes, and the laundry, and the homework and the science project.

We add more forms of communication: television, radio, email, Internet, regular mail, newspapers, magazines, cell phones, voicemail, text messaging.

More lives to keep track of, including people we don't even know. Pretty soon, there is no time and we are multi-tasking every task, including some that should be enjoyable.

We read while we eat, we talk while we drive, we work on three things at once. Simple pleasures are eroded by a sense of urgency and the need for more adrenalin to keep us going. No time to say, "Hello", "Goodbye".

Not only is productivity addicting, but so is the feeling of contributing – you know what you are doing and you are doing a good job, you can help someone else do a good job; you can right a wrong or save the world. "No one else can do as good a job as I", quickly morphs into everyone asking you for your input and assistance all the time. More work for you, you just took on their work.

We work this hard because our society sets up overwork as a model of success. "Supermoms", mandatory overtime, full-time students with full-time jobs.

One day I saw a 40-ish single mom who was working two jobs, going to school full-time and raising her children. She was exhausted, stressed, depressed, gaining weight and forgetting things.

"Why are you doing all of this", I asked.

"For my kids, so I can get a better job."

I looked at her without any humor, and replied, "If you live long enough".

We are operating at a level of INTENSITY that causes DISEASE.

We have lost our ability to play, and live and love. We have lost our ability to experience emotion because we are so busy working. We have lost the ability to relax, and think and be alone with ourselves. We have lost the ability to feel content with our circumstances. We have forgotten how to look at the sky and wonder about the stars.

We have lost the ability to experience emotion when we are under severe chronic stress.

Hard at work and numbed out to everything and everybody.

Here's the problem: If you don't allow your brain a chance to process your life experiences as they happen, the emotions will leak out anyway. You will be angry, and irritable, and depressed, and stressed and anxious, even when you don't want to be that way.

Which leads you directly to what I like to call "The Last Job". The job of suppressing your emotions so you can keep working an insane pace.

The reason that stress is so deadly is because the last job you take on is an impossible task. You may be able to do the laundry and your homework at the same time, you may be able to work all day, make dinner for the kids and go to school at night, but you cannot suppress normal emotion.

In order to keep up your pace, you must suppress the emotion or you will "break down". My office is filled with people who start the appointment by saying "I think I'm having a breakdown". "I feel like I'm losing my mind".

If you WORK to suppress unwanted emotions, you develop disease. You simply added more work and increased your stress level.

I am addicted to stress. Everywhere I look I see work that needs to be done, whether it's a book that needs writing or a counter that needs wiping. I cannot pet the dog without noticing a mat that needs combing. There will never be an end to this manuscript because I am forever editing. I can answer your questions, and their questions and everybody's questions no matter what I am doing and how exhausted I feel.

When it's time for me to relax and have fun, I often cannot. Unless I eat. Then I relax. The food pours out dopamine and GABA and serotonin and acetylcholine into my parched brain until I am positively serene. Am I relaxing because I'm healthy? Or am I relaxing because the food just drugged me into forgetting what I was doing

People are often sent to the psychiatrist for treatment of Depression when in fact they are shutting down due to overwhelming stress. They may be diagnosed as having Bipolar Disorder because they cannot sleep from their minds working all night. They may be diagnosed as having Attention Deficit Disorder because they have lost the ability to prioritize and organize because of overload.

The effects of stress can mimic psychiatric disorders, but they are not the same. Stress is a condition of overwork. Anxiety is a condition of fear. Depression is a condition of suffering. It is possible to have one or all of these simultaneously. The treatments may overlap, or may be different for each condition.

For the five or ten minutes that you are stress-eating, your brain is transported to a lower-stress zone. You give your body, your brain, and everyone else in your life a break from the jagged energy you are projecting.

If you are eating all the time in response to stress, "all the time" is simply a reflection of HOW STRESSED YOU ARE!

Stress-eating can also become your most effective DO NOT DISTURB sign, temporarily insulating you from further bombardment. Most people, even bosses and kids, will leave you alone while you are eating, even if it's just the amount of time it takes to eat a candy bar from a vending machine. The only other place to get this kind of peace is in the bathroom.

Boredom is also a type of stress.

Your brain asks you to feed yourself all the time. Sometimes it is asking for nutrients, real food, physical exercise, or love. Sometimes it is calling for brain exercise – YOUR BRAIN WANTS TO THINK!!! If you are bored silly, you will become stressed.

You can turn off your soul's request for learning and creativity with television or food. But you will not remove the drive to think and learn. You are born that way. Tomorrow if you are bored, you will go through the same struggle again.

Just in case you thought this was only about your own personal stress, there's more. You can also absorb other people's stress, particularly if they are close to you. Stressed people have a tendency to pour out their problems in rapid-fire succession, one after another, with great energy and emotion.

Your best friend comes over to tell you about all of her problems, and when she leaves you feel like you're on a trampoline, bouncing endlessly. You have now added your friend's stress to yours! It's like compounding interest on a loan; the balance due keeps going up!

One easy secret to prevent you from absorbing someone else's stress is to simply cross your arms in front of you while they are talking. By putting your arms over your heart, you have blocked their flow of stress from entering your body.

If you are overloaded with work, be honest with yourself. Decide if some of your deadlines are too grueling and can be extended or maybe even cancelled. Look around and see who can help you. Beware of using lack of money or time as an excuse to grind your health into illness.

Decide if some of the work you are doing is not really yours to do, have you taken on someone else's job?

Relief from stress is about learning to say no: no to demands, no to internal goals, no to family expectations, no to overzealous work projects. Saying no does not mean quitting your job in a bad economy, nor does it mean walking away from a difficult supervisor and getting fired. Saying no means acknowledging your physical and emotional limits and respecting them.

Relief from stress is about recognizing your body's signals. When you cannot sleep, and you cannot relax, and you cannot stop thinking about work, you are overworked.

The solution to stress and overwork lies in learning and practicing proper endings. To be able to say this is my workday and I am now off. This is my homework time and it is now over. The day's work has ended and this is my sleep time. This is my stress, and this is yours and I cannot accept it. These are boundaries, yours, mine, and ours.

The solution for stress is to recognize that for your body, rest is as essential as exercise.

For your brain, quiet is as vital as thinking.

For your spirit, solitude is as healing as company.

The solution to stress is to accept your humanity and all its limitations.

Chapter
5

Depression – Vital Exhaustion

*In the month before sudden death heart attacks,
some people experience "vital exhaustion", a fatigue
so profound that no amount of rest seems to help.
Depression is "vital exhaustion" of the mind.*

If you think of depression as a sound, it is the lowest sound you hear. It is the sound of exhaustion - mournful, deep, and echoing inside your being. It is so low a tone, you cannot sing it, but you know the feeling. It is a tone that is so low, you feel like you're underwater listening to it. Moving in slow motion. Drowning.

Depression has many faces, it fools patients and doctors alike.

Depression is a state of too little energy - the exact opposite of anxiety. Sit on the couch and watch television in the dark on a glorious sunny summer day when everyone else is outside having a great time. Too paralyzed to move. Too exhausted to sleep.

You say to yourself, "I'm going to get up and go out there, pretend I'm having a good time, and then maybe I'll feel better." But you never get up, you never move, and pretty soon it's Monday morning again and you have to go to work, the weekend is over and you never rested.

Depression may be a feeling of death, and darkness, and despair, and sadness, and hopelessness and rumination. It may be the constant mind-numbing litany in your brain of everything you've ever done wrong. For some people and in some cultures, depression is a physical sensation of heaviness and deep aching pain somewhere in your body.

Some people develop a higher energy depression filled with anger and irritability. They spend their relationships pushing away those they love and insulting those who love them. The hostility ensures they will be alone and lonely, with only their depression and pain to keep them company.

Depression can combine with anxiety, or substance abuse or physical illness - or all of the above.

Unlike anxiety, which is a state of constant motion, the hallmark of depression is paralysis. Even if the Garden of Eden is on the other side of your doorstep, and you can see the lushness and beauty and serenity, you still have to take a step forward to get there.

When you have horrible, crippling, vegetative depression, that step might as well be the Grand Canyon, and I might as well be asking you to fly.

In time, you develop automatic negative thoughts (ANTS). Every waking moment is a combination of impossibilities, victimization and pessimism. I can't. They won't. It will never happen. There's no way. They did it to me. You can feel yourself swimming in negativity, yet you are convinced that is the real version of the world.

Wait a minute. How can a low energy state produce an active busy mind? It doesn't. Your brain is not overly active, nor busy. It is repeating itself. Like the proverbial broken record. Same thought, over and over again. And you're exhausted listening to it. You are actually using less physical brain and less physical body when you are very depressed.

And if you stay at this level of depression for a long time, your memory actually shrinks, and so does your brain.

Here's the weird paradox of paralyzing depression – it's addicting. Just like food. No matter how horrible you feel, your brain has a comfort level set by familiarity. Chronic depression and despair begin to feel like home. You will automatically seek this familiar place in your mind – a kind of persistent grinding transmission that you become used to after awhile.

Our natural energies and emotions fluctuate within a range of comfortable energies. We become uncomfortable when we are out of our usual range. A mild mannered person who experiences rage becomes very uncomfortable. A depressed, despairing person is more comfortable in a familiar low range of unhappy feelings, EVEN THOUGH THEY ARE MISERABLE. We seek relief, but only a little bit at a time.

Your brain likes an easy, steady state of comfort. Which is why it takes WORK to move out of your depression.

It helps to picture yourself taking baby steps. If you feel despair, sadness will be an improvement. If you feel anger, irritability will be an improvement. In time, you will inch up to more pleasant states.

Depression does peculiar things to appetites. Some people cannot eat a bite and lose large amounts of weight. Even obese people can have this reaction of "failing to thrive". Others feed their depression with an endless intake of comfort foods. Some people alternate between the two, often not eating all day and bingeing on sweets at night.

A sneaky thing happens when a depressed person binges on carbohydrates. They feel better momentarily. A brain surge of serotonin, and GABA and acetylcholine. They relax, they sleep. Sugar becomes a sleeping pill, a nerve pill, and an energy pill.

What a great medication - for 20 minutes - except for the lingering side effects: mood swings, anger, irritability, worsening depression, brain fog, diabetes, heart disease, memory problems.

Comfort foods are most often sweet and/or dairy. Gallons of ice cream. I used to eat a pint of ice cream every night. No dinner, just ice cream. Years ago. Alone in my apartment. Too tired to cook, too depressed to stop and get something healthier. Just didn't care. And the ice cream, by virtue of the milk and sugar and chocolate, increased just enough serotonin that I was able to get up the next morning - sad, hopeless and swollen - and start the whole cycle again. After awhile, I switched to a box of cookies. Every night, the same brand. And after I got tired of that, I switched to chocolate candy.

On a health kick, I would eat pasta instead. To my brain, it was the same difference. Simple carbohydrates turn into sugar in the body. It just takes a few minutes longer.

I ate to shut off my mind and get some relief from the pain. I didn't care about my health or my body or my future. I was drowning.

BETTER LIVING THROUGH CHEMISTRY IS A NOT ENTIRELY TRUE

There isn't a magic pill for depression, although there are some very helpful traditional medications and psychotherapies as well as alternative treatments. Helpful, not curative. Yet depression can be cured; just not by medication alone.

In the world of medications for depression, a 30% decrease in symptoms is considered partial remission. Full remission is a 50% relief of symptoms. If you had cancer, you would not consider yourself in remission if you still had half or two-thirds of your disease present.

The expectation of most people when they take medication for depression is that the depression will GO AWAY.

The reality for most people is: with standard depression treatments, they will feel and function somewhat better – but not 100 percent. They can get out of bed, shower and maybe go to work or take care of their family or have a conversation with a stranger. That's a long way from feeling "happy".

Why don't the medications and treatments work fully to "cure" the depression?

Because, for most people, depression is not an exclusive chemical imbalance. Depression is an accumulation of relentless contributing factors such as psychosocial stressors, illness, diet, fatigue, genetics, and substance abuse. The end result of your body's stress management system gone awry. Overloaded, undersupplied, underpaid, overworked. Your brain cells just simply don't have enough materials to run your brain properly under the circumstances.

Medication can only do so much when you are having marital problems, or parenting problems, or problems at work, or lack of work, or lack of money, or drinking every night, or have chronic pain, or cannot sleep and cannot quiet your mind.

Here's what I learned...the depression NEVER got better from all that sugar, and carbohydrates and fat. IT JUST KEPT GETTING WORSE. And I just kept getting fatter and sicker. All of those foods, including all of the preservatives, contributed to much of my sadness and lack of energy and irritability. What I ate was making me worse. What would heal me was what I wasn't eating.

Many psychiatric medications can increase your appetite and increase your cravings for carbohydrates, particularly sweets.

You are not going to feel better when you gain another 60 pounds. If you are on any medications that have these side effects, discuss alternatives with your physician.

There is a war going on in your head. Your toxic, overfed, undernourished brain is mounting chemical warfare on your mood. Your greatest struggle with depression is not what you eat, but what you think. There is only you on both sides of the struggle.

Begin your recovery by RECOGNIZING that some of what you are thinking and saying is exaggerated and maybe even irrational. At the very least, it is repetitive.

The most effective way to break the habit of depression-thinking is to INTERRUPT automatic negative thoughts as they occur. CONSTANTLY. A thousand times an hour, in the beginning. Every waking moment. The simple act of recognizing, "uh-oh here I go again" successfully interrupts the negative thought. No catchy affirmations to substitute. You won't believe them anyway. With all that pain in your soul, positive thinking will sound false. Keep in mind your automatic negative thoughts are not universal truths, they are just habit.

Limit your exposure to negative thought makers such as violence, news stories, and heated arguments. They will always make you feel worse.

Several days after the 9-11 World Trade Center tragedy, I saw a young mother in a paralyzing depression. She had not moved from the television for four days. She was not caring for herself or her children, and could not stop crying. She had lost the will to live because of this terrible event. I had her estimate how many times she thought she had seen the airplanes crash and the twin towers of the World Trade Center crumble. 4,000 times. In less than four days.

I had to help her understand that it was okay to turn off the television. It was okay to eat, and sleep, and see sunshine and play with her kids. Continuing to enjoy her life did not dishonor those who died. They would likely not want her to die a sympathetic, withering death along with them.

Every time you feel badly, change something. Change the station. Walk away. Open the drapes. Drink tea instead of coffee. You'll feel better.

SYMPTOMS OF DEPRESSION

Depressed or irritable mood most of the day, nearly every day

Loss of interest in pleasurable life activities

Isolating from friends and family

Change in sleep and eating patterns

Change in Energy (too much or too little)

Fatigue or loss of initiative, loss of functioning

Constant feelings of worthlessness or guilt

Diminished ability to think or concentrate or make decisions

Thoughts that life is not worth living; wishing to die, thoughts of suicide

IF YOU ARE EXPERIENCING SYMPTOMS OF DEPRESSION, SEEK MEDICAL ATTENTION IMMEDIATELY.

YOU ARE NOT ALONE AND YOU DO NOT NEED TO SUFFER, TREATMENT IS AVAILABLE.

The National Suicide Hotline Numbers are Toll-Free and open every minute, of every day 24 hours / 7 days a week

1-800-SUICIDE (1-800-784-2433)

1-800-273-TALK (1-800-273-8255)

TTY: 1-800-799-4TTY (4889)

Chapter

6

Anxiety – I Can't Make It Stop

"Meanwhile, in the broad and lofty chamber set apart for occasions of import, the Abbot himself was pacing impatiently backwards and forwards, with his long white nervous hands clasped in front of him. His thin, thought-worn features and sunken, haggard cheeks bespoke one who had indeed beaten down that inner foe whom every man must face, but had none the less suffered sorely in the contest. In crushing his passions he had well-nigh crushed himself."

> — *Arthur Conan Doyle,*
> *The White Company (1891)*

"There is no writer's block. There is only fear."

> — *Mark David Gerson, The Voice of*
> *the Muse: Answering the Call to Write*

I had a full-blown panic attack when I was accepted into medical school. I was at work as a secretary in the Intensive Care Unit, watching the interns move between critically ill patients. I suppose I was imagining myself in their position, having to act fast to save lives, sometimes winning, sometimes losing, but I don't really remember what I was thinking. All of a sudden I had crushing chest pain and couldn't breathe. Sweat and tears were pouring out of me uncontrollably. I went down to the Emergency Department where the resident doctor checked my labs and electrocardiogram, pronounced my heart healthy, and informed me I was having a panic attack "with good reason".

It didn't resemble any version of anxiety I knew.

It resembled terror.

I had no conscious brain working. Nowhere to run, no trying to figure out how to escape the jaws of a circling shark. Only bodily sensation.

I couldn't get it to stop.

The most desperate patients I see are those who have relentless, unremitting anxiety and panic. I don't blame them. If depression is a state of near paralysis, anxiety is the exact opposite. It is a tornado of harmful energy inside you, screaming to get out. If you could reach inside your head and pull out your brain, you would.

The serious anxiety you experience might be coming from your biology. How do you know if you are genetically predisposed to anxiety?

Some folks are born with exaggerated "startle" reflexes. If you have an exaggerated startle, you are more likely to suffer from anxiety.

Determining who has an exaggerated startle reflex is easy. Imagine two kids comfortably lying down in the den, watching television, engrossed in a show. You want them to get up and get ready for dinner. You call them. No response. You call again. No response except the sound of the television. You're annoyed… you walk in the room and in your best drill sergeant voice, loud and sharp, you bark, "I SAID LET'S GO!!!!" … the kid who jumps a mile at the sound of your voice has the exaggerated startle.

The other kid didn't blink and is still watching television completely undisturbed.

Depression is a state of being imprisoned in the thoughts and memories of the past. Anxiety is the torture of imagined pain and fear in the future. Whereas your family and friends can help you identify the half-truths of depressive memory, no one can entirely dismiss a sense of foreboding as unrealistic. Who knows when lightning will strike?

Meanwhile, you are left with a miserable droning in your brain, a feeling of wanting to jump out of your skin. You can't sleep. When you do sleep, you dream of taking an exam without studying, or being naked in a crowd; your stomach aches, your chest hurts, you can't breathe. That amount of EXTRA energy does not help you function, it PREVENTS you from focusing on anything else. YOU ARE AFRAID.

Eventually, it burns the life out of you. All that extra energy you had turns into exhaustion, and begins to look a lot like depression.

Eating makes the anxiety better temporarily. Your brain floods with feel-good chemicals like GABA and acetylcholine and for a few moments, you're not as panicked.

I have a recurring pattern of anxiety that overtakes me anytime I have a goal. I spend hours frenetically chasing my soul before I can get started. When I eat, the anxiety may leave, but unfortunately, the goal also disappears. I am left sleeping on the couch, with a half box of cookies and an extra pound, hours of time playing solitaire, a sick disappointed feeling, disrupted sleep and mood, and the unwanted loss of my passion.

Every time I sat down to write a page or a chapter in this book, the buzzing would start and I wanted to go eat - anything, as fast as I could. I tried putting my laptop on a table on the treadmill, figuring I could walk off some of the extra energy. I tried playing calming music, inspiring tapes, meditating. Maybe the anxiety was a little less at times, but mostly the call to food was greater than the call to the pen.

I didn't understand what was happening to me. The expert psychiatrist. Why was I unable to stop the fear and procrastination that gripped me?

One day I did an assisted meditation, one that adds light or sound or movement to help quiet the mind enough to overcome internal chatter and ask a question.

Why do I have such bad writer's block? Why am I so anxious?

In my meditation, inspiration flowed freely into my head. Until it slammed directly into a block of pure anxiety in the center of my brain.

I was scared. Scared I would fail. Scared I would succeed. Scared that everything and nothing would change. Scared of the task. Scared of the results.

I was doing this to myself.

I was so scared that the flow of creative joy that ached to travel through me was blocked.

The creative energy wanted to travel THROUGH ME. Not from me.

The word "conduit" echoed in my mind.

I saw the block evaporate and the golden creative light flow freely from above, into my mind and out my fingers onto the keyboard.

These are not my words, These are the words of a greater source. I am not alone in what I try to do. After that, the writers block was gone. It comes back at times, but I know what to do.

The answer to anxiety is TRUST.

Trust that you are not alone. Trust that you will be fine. Trust that your purpose is achievable. Trust that you will find the help you need to continue. Trust that if you fall, someone or something will catch you. Trust that even if the person you think should catch you fails, someone else will. The odds are in your favor – the lightning will miss.

Trust that even the mistakes you make have meaning. And that somehow they contribute to your greater purpose. Even if, at this moment, you don't understand how this is possible.

Most behavioral health providers will tell you to meditate or do guided imagery for your anxiety. That's great – except for two minor problems. If you have constant anxiety, it will be nearly impossible to quiet down your mind enough to do the meditation. Unless you eat first. Plus meditation takes too long. Anxiety and Attention Deficit Disorder have a lot in common – people are impatient and hyperactive with the attention span of a gnat.

You might be experiencing serious anxiety for an acute medical reason. Your blood sugar could be too low or too high. Your thyroid might be on overdrive. You may have an abnormal heartbeat. Persistent, unrelenting anxiety needs to be checked out medically.

It might be stress-related, environmental or toxic, dietary (such as too much caffeine or sugar or not enough protein), not enough sleep, or too much noise. It might be medication or substance withdrawal – if you use pain pills, or alcohol, or marijuana, or benzodiazepines or the computer all the time. The anxiety sensation that some people experience after starting on anti-depressants comes from serotonin EXCESS. Those people describe feeling WORSE after starting medication, not better.

Do not accept that your anxiety is psychological until you have ruled out all other sources, including your diet and environment.

When I recently had palpitations and hair loss, it turned out to be mercury toxicity from a cracked metal filling rather than thyroid, or cardiac or panic as I first suspected. Thanks to Mark Hyman, M.D., author of The UltraMind Solution, I was able to identify a possible cause of these symptoms and work with my doctor to test and resolve the problem. (I had my wisdom teeth out at the tender age of 54!)

Change your diet to include more foods that
promote GABA and acetylcholine production
in the brain, and add relaxation and music
that quiets you. Talk to your physician about
medications that may be inadvertently
increasing your anxiety.

The secret to decreasing anxiety is this…ALL THE TIME. You are anxious *all the time*, therefore you must use every tool to interrupt the anxiety *all the time*. The first time you experience real relaxation, the kind that shoots out relaxation chemicals (acetylcholine) from your vagus nerve, the kind that washes your insides so you feel like a baby blanket of Jell-O™, you'll be hooked. The good news is that the more you do your relaxation, the more your anxiety will decrease. And the more you relax, the more ADDICTED you will become to relaxing.

The second secret to decreasing anxiety is to add movement. You will be worse trying to hold a yoga pose, like trying to keep a lid on an overfilled pot. Walk, do tai chi, tap your foot, sing, dance, do anything you can to dissipate the extra energy while you are acutely anxious, then allow your body to slow down at its own pace.

The more you relax naturally, the less you will eat.

From Master Chunyi Lin (Spring Forest Qi Gong):

When you feel overwhelmed with too much energy it generally means you have too much energy in your head. Try this technique: drop your shoulders, place your hands on your belly button and take long gentle deep breaths. Dropping your shoulders is very important - actually it's a trick. Remember to drop your shoulders.

When having an anxiety attack drink a glass of cold water, take long gentle deep breaths, step outside and get some fresh air and try not to focus on that emotion. Instead, feel how good you feel.

Chapter

7

Anger – Feeding the Fire
Inside and Out

"In the beginning the Universe was created.
This has made a lot of people very angry and
has been widely regarded as a bad move."

— *Douglas Adams*

Anger can lead us to the verge of being irrational. We are an angry world. We are an angry society. We are angry people. We feed our souls with angry thoughts and stories. We are used to being angry.

We are so angry that we are on the brink of destroying our selves and our planet. From our anger!

Now, that's IRRATIONAL.

Anger is a higher energy state than depression, easier to tolerate than depression. When you are angry, you move. You take deep breaths. You think rapidly. You make decisions easily.

Anger feels much better to you; it just doesn't feel better to everyone else.

Here is the truth of anger: We are angry because WE LIKE THE WAY IT FEELS. It makes us feel strong. God help us.

Anger used as motivation for change can save the world. Anger turned into hatred and resentment can destroy the world. When you create strong energy directed farther outward, you can ultimately harm EVERYONE, including yourself.

The power of anger is so strong it can change your heart. And it certainly can change someone else's.

I once watched a man in the Cardiac Intensive Care Unit change his heart rhythm when his detested daughter-in-law walked into the room. He was sitting in bed comfortably chatting with the medical team. His family entered the room. As soon as he saw his daughter-in-law, his eyes turned into laser beams and he started screaming profanities at her. In a nanosecond, his heart rhythm flipped from normal sinus rhythm into an abnormal dangerous fibrillation. The heart monitor alarmed emergently.

Wow, we said, as we moved into action, he must really hate her.

He hated her so much it almost cost him his life.

Fat people are some of the angriest people I know. I know that because I am one of those chronically angry people.

When I am really, really hungry, I turn into a raving maniac.

This morning I had two hours of business meetings. I didn't start the morning feeling angry, but I did walk into those meetings feeling stressed, pressured for time, and overloaded with too many urgent things to do.

I hadn't had enough sleep.

I didn't have time for breakfast.

I didn't have time for tai chi and stretching.

My back hurt.

Bad combination.

Hungry, stressed, tired and in pain.

By the time the first hour ended, I was visibly angry. My passion about the topic had crossed the line from strong feeling into the realm of irrationality. Fortunately, not into the insanity zone (yet). I had become the kind of raging person about whom people say, "What is her problem?"

Which means, I went into the second hour with a giant chip on my shoulder. Not a good way to start a problem solving session.

In the meantime, something interesting occurred.

I was so angry, I was no longer tired.

I was not hungry.

I didn't have any pain.

I was thriving on the stress and looking for more. "Loaded for bear", as people say, gunning for a fight.

I was operating on pure adrenalin. For no good reason other than I skipped breakfast, and missed exercising and was a little tired.

Every cell in my body was working full speed. I had more energy than I knew what to do with. That excess of physical energy was clearly impairing my good judgment and my ability to effectively communicate. But boy, could I type fast. Or drive fast. Or talk fast.

Of course, no one in the meetings was listening to me because my tone and my stance overpowered my words. They saw the movie; they didn't have the sound on because the volume was too loud.

I'd like to be able to say that I didn't ruin their day. But I know I did. Anger steams out of a person and scalds everyone within shouting distance. I ruined many hours, even if it was only temporary. What happens to people who live or work with an angry person day after day? They get scalded. And they feel pain.

After awhile, I calmed myself down. My friends and husband calmed me down. My coworkers calmed me down.

I ate food. I took a few minutes of quiet time.

I reassessed my life in three deep breaths and asked myself, "Do I want my insides to boil and explode, or do I want to live in harmony with all of the beauty and goodness around me and quit acting like an ass?" It took an extra two breaths to decide, because all that energy actually felt pretty good.

Finally it was over.

It was the psychological equivalent of a thunderstorm. It wasn't a tornado, there was no permanent damage, but I had a little cleaning-up to do. I had to apologize to people about being angry for no good reason.

Salty crunchy food cravings are often the result of anger and frustration. Move away from table salt toward sea salt. Add hot and spicy to your craving food – eat spicy dips such as salsa or guacamole and put Tabasco or peppers on your meal. Think of forest firefighters. When they want to "break" a forest fire, they set a smaller controlled burn to stop the bigger one from progressing.

If you feel anger, eating hot and spicy food will cause your brain to release calming endorphins. Before you punch a wall, eat a jalapeno. The fire in your mouth will put out the fire in your brain.

One of the experiences that obese individuals have when they lose large amounts of weight is the discovery of hidden, unexpressed anger and rage. The food has acted as an effective anti-anger medication all these years.

I can't be angry right now because I'm stuffed and sleepy and can't move.

Unfortunately, the food you choose may actually be making the anger worse after you consume it. Large amounts of unhealthy foods can cause wild fluctuations in blood sugar or brain chemicals or can cause a person to feel like they are in withdrawal.

A bag of crunchy chips may stop the rage, but the next day, the fluid retention and swollen feeling will have you swimming in irritability. Here you go again.

Calming energy does not extinguish high-energy righteous anger. To put out the fire of anger, substitute other high-energy states. Exercise is one. Dancing. Talking. Use that energy for expression and health.

Go to a gym and lift weights, mow the lawn, punch a punching bag. Work your energy until you are physically tired and your body starts to relax and release some of that anger-energy.

The true antidote to anger is compassion. I can hear the groans now. Another forgiveness lecture.

Hear me out.

The antidote to anger is compassion FOR YOURSELF.

I am not telling you anger is a bad thing. I am telling you that anger is a form of stress that can be very harmful to your body, your self-esteem, your weight and your relationships.

We are energy beings in an energy universe. When I erupt in uncontrolled energy, I feel it. You feel it. I absorb it. You absorb it. We both suffer.

If you are angry, take a minute and feel kindness toward yourself. You have had to deal with so much pain, and difficulty and unfairness in the world. You're stressed, you're exhausted, you're overworked. You're undervalued. You're underpaid. You're disrespected. You may have been abused and discriminated against. No wonder you're so angry. If you can allow some compassion for yourself, you will feel your heart start to soften. And that's all it takes for the anger to begin to dissipate. It's not worth having a heart attack over.

And then you won't eat as much. Today.

Chapter

8

The Black Hole of Trauma

Here's the chapter I was most afraid to write. Everyday for years I have worked with patients who are severely traumatized, and I see what trauma does to hearts and minds and souls and bodies. This is not my story, but it might be yours.

What could I ever write that would adequately and accurately represent the traumatized obese patient?

One day I got into a taxi driven by a very nice talkative older man. He told me about his family, he told me about his retirement, he told me about the night all the surviving members of his infantry unit were killed by a drunk driver while they were on their way home after 2 years in the infantry in World War II. In graphic detail. Five minutes after I got into the cab. Not knowing who I was.

While my cousin painted the living room walls, he told my one year old niece about the selection line for the gas chambers in the concentration camp. It didn't matter that she wasn't listening and couldn't understand. It was where his mind was on a beautiful summer day half a century later.

That is the trauma survivor. Years later and it's still the first thing on their minds. Every moment of life that came after that trauma is secondary.

The easiest way to explain trauma to someone who has never experienced it, is to compare it to the "music worm" in your head. You know the silly jingle that someone starts singing and you can't get it to stop in your mind?

Now imagine if the sounds and images and smells and thoughts that you have in your head are gruesome. And you can't get them to stop.

That is the experience of trauma.

Trauma turns a full soul into a skeleton. Some people are able to compartmentalize their trauma, they file it away in some cabinet in their mind and only open the drawers once in a great while. Those folks do better overall, they are able to participate in life's goodness.

Other people have their trauma strewn all over the rooms of their brain, and there's nowhere to turn in their head to avoid the memories. Including sleep. They need something to numb the images that are constant. That is the obese trauma patient.

Overeating numbs the feelings, fades the memories, distances the anger.

If I had been horribly traumatized, I would want to eat all the time to make the memories stop.

Successful treatment of trauma patients involves re-integration of their body, mind and spirit. They are in pieces. There is no wholeness, no start to finish, no uninterrupted timeline.

There is before the trauma. Then there is the trauma. There may never be an "after" the trauma.

All of the work that people do in therapy to compartmentalize and reframe the trauma is designed to move present life up into the forefront and the trauma back into second place. We never try to get people to forget the trauma. It's not possible.

Your body remembers the trauma even when your mind does not. Maybe even your cells remember.

Years ago, I had a plane crash survivor in the Intensive Care Unit with multiple fractures. He was on a rotating bed so that his weight was evenly distributed along his skeleton. Mostly he slept in a lightly anesthetized state. But once every few hours, when his center of gravity shifted into the position he experienced in the crashing plane, he awoke and started screaming. His body remembered even while his mind was asleep.

I once saw a young, otherwise healthy, woman with throat cancer. The typical person who gets throat cancer is an elderly man with a lifetime of drinking and smoking. I wondered how it came to be that a non-smoking, non-drinking young woman with no family history of this awful disease developed throat cancer. "Oh, that's easy", she said. "My mother used to beat me and I always wanted to scream at her, but I never did". Her throat remembered the sensation, even when her mind no longer thought about it.

My office is filled with people who have experienced physical, sexual, emotional trauma. Sometimes the trauma is not theirs directly; it is someone they love dearly who has suffered. The image of their loved one suffering is unimaginable horror. The effects can be almost identical.

And it doesn't have to be life-threatening. It only has to be life-altering for a person to be traumatized. Bullying, child molestation, date rape, cancer and medical treatment all fall into this category where an event or events forever change a person's life and how they view themselves.

When we feel badly, we revert to the comfort foods of our childhood. We saw from the public's response to food after the terrorist attacks on September 11th that the demand for junk food such as ice cream and chips rose 12% (AC Nielson survey). I wonder what happened to macaroni and cheese sales.

I know this. Eating does not heal trauma. Ever.

Art heals trauma sometimes

Love heals trauma sometimes

Prayer heals trauma sometimes

Telling your story heals trauma sometimes

Being with people who understand you heals sometimes.

My reason for being here might be because I am the one who will bear witness to the story of your trauma. If you can do that for someone else, they will begin to heal from their trauma. Sometimes.

Chapter 9

On Dying, Grief And Eating: The Abyss of Emptiness

"There are things that we don't want to happen but have to accept, things we don't want to know but have to learn, and people we can't live without but have to let go."

— *Author Unknown*

It is the purpose and work of being human to experience emotion. Our nervous systems are programmed this way. We love, we laugh, we anger, we suffer and we grieve. Wise humans learn that over time, if left alone, emotions will change like everything in nature. Even the strongest, most desolate of emotions will shift. Sometimes we need help getting through the storms, but if we can hold on long enough, the storm will break.

I am a spontaneous griever. I cry when someone dies whom I've never met. I cry when someone is harmed even though I know they will survive. I weep over the stories in the newspaper, the radio, the Internet and greeting cards. I cry over wars, and crimes, and oppression and history. Sometimes I cry when patients talk. There's nothing to medicate away. This is not abnormal. It is my soul telling me that I am witnessing something profound. My tears have become my reality check.

I am also a grief eater. Grief opens up a hole inside of me that no amount of food can fill. It's as if my appetite is connected to my heart instead of my stomach. When my beloved childhood dog died, I gained 20 pounds. The aching emptiness was intolerable. When my friend moved away, I gained 10 pounds. When my beloved grandmother died, I gained 20 pounds. When my mother died, I gained 40 pounds. In between these losses, I would recover and lose a little weight (usually not all) until the next grief cycle began. Then came, what was for me the mother of all grief, when I realized I would not be a mother myself, I gained (and then failed to lose) 60 pounds. Until, once again, I healed.

I can trace my weight gains in chunks based on who died, who left, and who was never born. I can trace my grief to separations from people and places I loved: the last day of camp or the last day of elementary school - leaving someone or someplace I loved, or a stage of my life that was ending.

I can trace my weight gains to anticipating grief, experiencing grief, and reliving grief.

I can trace my failure to drop weight to continual cycles of grief.

And here's what I know about eating for grief. It didn't help. Not one chocolate bar, not one binge, not one pizza. None of it helped at all. The grief stayed. Maybe for a few minutes while I had some extra serotonin and dopamine and oxytocin from all that food flooding my brain, I didn't feel like dying, but within 30 minutes, the relief was gone.

I didn't get any more relief from the food than I would have gotten from a 20 minute walk with the dogs, or meditation or lavender bath.

And I didn't get anywhere near the amount of relief I would have gotten if I had just simply allowed myself to grieve. In a very spiritual way. On a very natural timetable. For as long as it took.

It is a solitary action. To heal from grief, you must converse with your feelings alone. You can do this in the company of others who respect your needs, in church, in the park, at the cemetery or at home. You can talk to yourself. You can talk to your loved one who died. You can talk to God. You can listen to music. You can be in silence and talk to no one.

Grieving is a full-time job. If you work 40 hours a week, you will feel as if you are working 80 hours. If you work 80 hours, you will need to make some time for yourself to grieve or rest or you may become ill. If you try to deny or suppress the tears, you will become ill. Heartsick. Broken-hearted. In Eastern medicine, the pancreas is the organ of joy. Disease in the pancreas occurs when people are unable to experience joy and happiness. They are depressed. They are grief-stricken.

There is no pill for grief and even if there was, I'm not sure I would prescribe it. When people come in my office and describe their loss, their love, their inability to wrap their arms around the physical being of a loved one, I ask them the same question, "Can you feel him or her around you?"

"Yes", say some. "I've never told anyone. The lights flickered, there was a scent, I felt their presence. I saw something. She came into my dream and it was as if she was standing there."

These people are the lucky ones. They have established a continuation of a cherished relationship without a physical presence.

I am one of those people who believe there is spiritual life after physical death. I believe that those who have died are joyful and can reach out to us at any time. My struggle was never about whether my loved ones who died were in a good place. My struggle was with my own grief. At times it was so thick that no one could communicate with me. Not in person and not in spirit.

Whether or not you believe in life-after-death is not essential. It does not take a feeling of your loved one's presence to heal from grief.

If the grief is too thick, if it encases a person in a dense blackness that cannot be penetrated, no memory can come through. No spiritual being can communicate. No love from those around you can comfort you.

There isn't a right or wrong way to grieve, and there isn't a way to speed up the process.

There is only healing.

Healing from grief comes in many forms – memories, dreams, thoughts, tears, wishes, and feelings.

How do you know the difference between Grief and Depression?

Grief comes in waves, often when you least expect it. I tell people to keep tissues in their car. When they start to drive, the part of their brain that usually works to maintain emotional composure is now busy driving and cannot do both simultaneously. Expect to cry when you drive or operate heavy machinery.

Depression sits like lead. Grief allows you to laugh. Depression has you thinking about yourself. Grief has you thinking about the person you lost.

A week after my mother died, I was on a plane to California. The in-flight movie was my mom's favorite comedy, and the lady in the row in front of me was a family friend I had known my whole life. I laughed and cried throughout the movie, and conversed with her old friend and enjoyed every minute of that plane ride. My mother was there, and I was never alone.

The natural course of an episode of uncomplicated Major Depression is approximately one year.

Grief can last months to years for a close family member, and 10 years or more for a child or a traumatic loss.

American culture wrongly expects rapid recovery from grief. Somewhere in our collective "un"wisdom, we decided grief was a process that lasts a few months. I have encountered people who experienced the death of a child and were asked by some clueless individual "It's been almost a year, aren't you over that by now?"

It is not natural to be separated from those we love. You will never be "over" it. Nor should you be. The depth of your grief is a reflection of the grandeur of your love for that person. Cherish that relationship.

Healing from grief is about finding a new dimension to an old relationship. The person you love, the place you lived, or the pet you had may be gone, but the experience you had with that beloved, and how you have changed as a result of that relationship, are with you forever.

Tim Russert, the famous journalist who died this year, guided me through this chapter. Whether he was really here in spirit or in my imagination is of no relevance. What is relevant is that his image sustained me through this very difficult chapter, which I had been avoiding. I wrote this the day Walter Cronkite died. They were our teachers.

They were the witness bearers to our grief. When we could not find words to express our sadness, they spoke simply and eloquently about being human. No matter what the loss, they maintained their composure and they gave us a framework for how to mourn. We were no longer alone, weeping in front of a television set. We were grieving together.

The healing of grief takes place alone among company.

Their memory and all of the caretakers of grief in the universe helped me write this chapter. The words flow, the tears flow, the feeling is real. I remember what I want to include, I organize without difficulty, I honor those whose memories I hold dear, and whose shoulders I ride upon. Without their collective wisdom, I know nothing. Without their collective love, I am alone.

This is healing.

Section Two

Counterfeit Energy:
Can Food Actually Keep Your Engine Running?
The Last Chance Surgeries
Somewhere Over The Rainbow:
Disconnected From Your Inner Self

Chapter

10

Counterfeit Energy: Can Food Actually Keep Your Engine Running?

The story of the body and obesity is the story of an automobile being run into the ground. At some point, it stops running. Things start breaking down; major repairs are required. Eventually it can't be fixed.

This is your body when you are obese.

Obesity is physically excruciating. Our bodies are not designed to carry around two or three times our body weight. Remember those old movie images of the slaves building the pyramids and carrying around huge stones on their backs, bent over and struggling from the weight? Only with obesity, you can't set it down anywhere. The huge weight stays with you. As a result, the story of obesity is pain, exhaustion and brain fog.

Can't move

Too tired

Too much pain

Can't remember

Exhausted means a lot of things – it may mean you need sleep, feel weak, cannot think clearly, run out of energy quickly. Fat people are exhausted. I was exhausted, you are exhausted, your friends and family and employers know that you are exhausted.

Fortunately, most exhaustion is not a sign of serious illness. In obese people, it is more often caused by one of the following four problems:

- Not getting enough quality sleep
- Eating the wrong foods, eating too much or too little food
- Not getting enough exercise
- Stress

I started my medical career as a surgical resident at a dynamic busy hospital. We routinely worked 100+ hours per week, stayed up all night, missed meals, and ran ourselves ragged in the old medical tradition. We never thought twice about being hungry or tired when someone's life was at stake. Still, even though we were young and driven, we were only human. The stress and exhaustion were relentless and took their toll on all of us.

To keep going, we lived on coffee, sugar-free colas and candy bars. We created a system of COUNTERFEIT ENERGY to keep us moving and thinking. My personal system consisted of sugar, caffeine, stress and anger. As long as I had an endless supply of those ingredients, I was good to go for another 18 hours. Despite the fact that those ingredients were injuring my brain, making it harder to think and act, and causing disease in my body.

Throwing sugar and caffeine in a body's fuel tank to get moving only works for about 20 minutes. Soon, the side effects take over. The body creates massive inflammation and fatigue as a result of an abnormal sugar and toxic load. Quickly we needed more sugar and caffeine because we become exhausted and sore again.

If you are exhausted, you may have an underactive thyroid, have diabetes or high blood pressure, rheumatological disease, heart or lung disease or any myriad of ailments that plague both obese patients and all of Western culture. Exhaustion can also be a side effect of certain medications used to treat these conditions.

Exhaustion may even be a forewarning of death. There is a syndrome called "Vital Exhaustion" that can precede sudden cardiac death for a month or more. In this type of exhaustion, people are unable to feel better no matter what changes they make.

Therefore, exhaustion ALWAYS needs to be checked out by a medical doctor before you begin a process of self-treatment for one simple reason – all of the self-treatment in the world will not have an impact if the reason you are exhausted is due to illness or medication.

Exhaustion can also occur when your energy is stolen, rather than used up.

For some people, the problem is not that you are using up your precious energy too quickly, or that you are not using good quality fuel to make energy. Sometimes, the people you love, the people you work with, the people and events you think about, are draining your energy. *They're sucking the life right out of you.*

Psychiatrist Judith Orloff M.D. calls these people, places and things *"energy vampires"*. People and situations that drain your vitality and leave you feeling helpless.

You know these folks. You start the conversation feeling fine, and you finish the conversation exhausted, irritable, and overwhelmed. Soon, you dread the interactions. After awhile, as a measure of self-preservation, you start to avoid them.

Lifelong obese people are particularly susceptible to energy vampires because we are reluctant to say no to people. We don't want to push anyone away. We absorb their bad energy, and then we eat to relieve ourselves of the symptoms WE get because of THEIR bad energy.

It doesn't start out that way. These are people you care about, share life events with, work with, live next door to. You start out wanting to have a satisfying two-way relationship with them.

I will share with you one of the earliest lessons for every mental health professional. You can't help everyone. Not everyone wants your help.

Some people are most comfortable existing with a fixed amount of unhappiness. If you attempt to help them, they will find something else in their lives in order to keep their unhappiness at their chosen level. The same applies to chaos and drama. Just when you think one catastrophe is averted, the person creates another.

If you are always available to absorb someone else's problems, you will never have energy or time to deal with your own.

It is not easy to learn how to set limits and tell people that you cannot help them at any given moment. If you have established yourself as the only person who can help your family and friends, you pay a large price for a fleeting sense of importance.

The first action you take to set limits with someone who is draining your energy for their own purposes is to recognize that you MUST TAKE CARE OF YOURSELF FIRST.

Rather than create more drama by confronting the individual, just simply start to protect yourself. Step your level of attention back a bit, shorten the amount of time, change the subject, fold your arms in front of you.

Imagine this person draining your energy and now imagine yourself cutting off the energy leak.

We are all connected, but we exist as individuals so that we may fulfill our own potential. We each have unique struggles and life stories to write. Lend a helping hand when you are able, and recognize that sometimes people have to help themselves.

Chapter

11

The Last Chance Surgeries

Modern medicine has found a way to cure obesity and diabetes. It involves surgically detouring your intestines or changing your stomach's food storage capacity, but at least you will finally be cured of overeating. Unless, you're not.

When bariatric surgery is successful, patients can lose hundreds of pounds and completely rewrite their futures. They can be cured of their diabetes, high blood pressure and high cholesterol, and begin to live life as healthier, more active individuals.

Bariatric surgeries are not without risk and complication, however, and require ongoing medical management following surgery with an experienced provider. Prospective bariatric surgery patients must be carefully screened for their ability to follow through with requirements. Patients may develop nutritional deficiencies, many patients gain weight back, some never really lose much weight. About one-third of patients develop subsequent addiction to some other substance besides food.

Patients often tell me that they look forward to the day when they will no longer be able to binge, no longer able to overeat, no longer able to eat sweets, ever again.

Unfortunately, it doesn't always work that magically. Bariatric surgery patients often believe that because many of them will experience "dumping syndrome" after eating a high carbohydrate meal, they will never be able to eat those foods again. Dumping syndrome is a kind of instant or slightly delayed diarrhea cleanse that is both unpleasant and guilt alleviating. The truth is that many patients eventually figure out how to consume calorie rich sweets and fats (usually in smaller quantities) and avoid the 'dumping syndrome'. They may not be able to eat an entire gallon of ice cream in one sitting, but they can certainly eat the gallon bite by bite over the course of one day. And your body doesn't know the difference.

Years ago, I had a bariatric surgery psychiatry patient who had successfully lost 250 pounds following surgery. He was a young man who developed a heart condition due to his obesity; for him, this surgery was a life-saver. One day I received a call that he needed to see me immediately. I had seen him just five weeks earlier and he had been fine, so I was concerned since this was clearly a change. The change was noticeable when he walked in the door. In one month he had gained almost 50 pounds.

"What happened?" I asked.

"I got dumped."

It was the kind of "dumping" syndrome that any of us can experience, the loss of a love. For this man, he resumed his binging within the parameters of his surgical stomach and intestinal capacity. And he gained 1/5 of his lost weight back within a few weeks.

Many bariatric patients will tell you that it isn't hard to regain most or all of the weight, even with a stomach the size of a thumb… that stretches to a pear, that easily holds half of a high fat, high sugar, high calorie lunch, and allows you to eat the other half later.

If you are a candidate for weight loss surgery, or if you have already had surgery, understand that your medical providers want you to be successful. All of us want you to lose weight, feel good, and heal.

In this book, you have learned some of the reasons why your brain is under attack.

If you have bariatric surgery, you will add the risk of nutritional deficiencies due to changes in your intestinal absorption.

Your body will feed your brain first before it feeds any other part of you. If you feel lethargic, or depressed or irritable, and you have had surgery or some other severe restriction of your food intake, or you are eating poor quality, low nutrient foods, you may be experiencing micronutrient deficiencies. Talk to your physician.

Bariatric surgery may cure your diabetes; it will not give you more money to pay the bills.

Bariatric surgery may help you lose 100 pounds or more; it will not relieve your stress at work, at home or in school.

Bariatric surgery may help you move around in society more easily, fit in chairs, and be more welcomed by strangers; it will not solve difficult family relationships.

Bariatric surgery may help you feel more attractive; it will not heal a broken soul.

If you are a bariatric surgery patient, understand that if you DO NOT learn to manage the emotional component to your eating, your results will be compromised. You might not lose as much weight as you planned. You might gain weight back. You might never really lose any weight.

You might become an alcoholic, start smoking, become addicted to pain medications, or gambling, or pornography or shopping.

This is not because you are a failure at bariatric surgery.

This is because your brain is screaming for more 'feel good' chemicals.

You are considering having weight-loss surgery, or have already had the surgery, because your physical health has deteriorated. The surgery is only one-third of the recovery; your psyche and your soul make up the other two-thirds. You have gone to all of this effort to preserve your body. Make room in your schedule for the health of your mind and your soul as well.

Chapter

12

Somewhere Over The Rainbow: Disconnected From Your Inner Self

(This chapter is dedicated to Israel "IZ" Kamakawiwo'ole)

"How do I know the ways of all things at the beginning? I look inside myself and see what is within me."

> — *21st verse, Tao Te Ching*
> *(with thanks to Dr. Wayne Dyer)*

"And as soon as my left hemisphere says to me "I am," I become separate. I become a single solid individual, separate from the energy flow around me and separate from you."

> — *Dr. Jill Bolte Taylor*
> *(www.TED.com) -TEDTALKS on*
> *A Stroke of Insight)*

Even if you do the work of emotion, even if you recover from grief and anger and depression, even if you start to move a little and nourish your body a little, even if you start to relax and gain some balance, you may still experience an overwhelming desire to eat.

Why do some people gain 100 pounds and others gain 500 pounds?

We see people in the news with extreme obesity. We see rescue efforts, medical efforts, and family interventions with bedridden, seriously ill people weighing hundreds and hundreds of pounds, sometimes a thousand. And sometimes we see a few amazing stories of superhuman weight loss.

I have had patients referred to me in this condition. They don't seem any different from other overweight people. They don't seem any different than I do. They laugh, they talk, they cry. They relate to the usual mundane activities. I medicate them, I work with them. They are not resistant to medical and psychological intervention. Despite my best efforts, I have not been able to reach any of them with any technique.

One day when I was outlining this book, I heard a beautiful rendition of "Somewhere Over The Rainbow", the Judy Garland song from the *Wizard of Oz*. I had heard this version once before on an episode of the television program *ER*. It was a soft, soulful rendition that brought tears to my eyes.

I had no idea who the singer was.

I found the funeral video of "Brudda IZ" Israel Kamakawiwo'ole, the 775-pound Hawaiian hero, an icon of island music, who died at the age of 38 from complications of obesity. His body lay in state in the capitol building in Hawaii. Thousands of people celebrated his life as they scattered his ashes in the Pacific Ocean.

The video showed this huge man with this little ukulele and a sweet clear tenor voice. In three minutes of song, he took the meaning of a homesick little girl's wish and transformed it into a belief that there was a better life some other time, some other place, somewhere over a rainbow.

As I watched, a feeling of unimaginable desperation and desolation washed over me. It was the most awful feeling I have ever had. It was clearly not simple grief.

It was a feeling of absolute and utter disconnectedness from my soul.

If I had that feeling, I would do anything I could to make it stop -
including eating until I weighed 800 pounds.

Our longest and deepest relationship is with our
body.

**If you treated your friends and family the
way you treat your body, you would lose them
all.**

Here's the scary part. Not only are you
treating your own body bad, you are treating the
bodies of your kids, and pets, and families, and
friends badly, too. No wonder there are so many
depressed, exhausted, irritable people out there.
Now I'm going to relieve a little bit of blame from
you, and place it squarely on the food industry.

In order to accomplish the goals of enticing
you with cheap, easy, irresistible foods, the
food industry makes food tastier with improved
texture by substituting laboratory chemicals for
food. Tastes better, though.

There are almost 3,000 artificial additives in
food. Every time you eat or drink something that
has a name you cannot spell, every time you
cannot picture that ingredient in your mind's
eye, you have ingested poison. The more toxic
food and drink you ingest, the harder your body
has to work to clear it out. If you eat and drink
only junk food everyday for years and years, your
brain and body are losing the battle and you are
developing illness.

We could talk about IZ, who lost his father and his brother, and how
he became a storyteller of Hawaiian people's oppression. We could talk

about how he had poor eating habits and the genetics for obesity. We could talk about how he had a great sense of humor, and related easily to others and how everyone loved him.

He knew how to help, how to laugh, how to work, how to inspire, how to love.

He knew how to exist in society, in family, in friendship.

He knew how to create.

He did not know how to co-exist with his innermost self.

We are all spiritual beings in physical bodies. Whether or not you believe in God or eternity does not matter. What matters is that you understand that you are MORE than your physical self. You are a song, and a prayer, and a tear and more. You are original thought. You are a creator. You love, you learn. These are not physical traits. The state of your physical being does not change these truths.

As an energy being, you can never be alone. You can never be disconnected from the flow of the universe. Every religion, every philosophy teaches this concept. Even the most devout atheist recognizes that there is energy of existence that is natural and indefinable, and runs through all living things.

Imagine how awful you would feel if you did not believe you were part of that energy. Imagine how desolate you would feel if you could not believe you were part of the universe.

I am not a religious leader or a philosopher. I am an observer and a healer.

Our health and well-being is a reflection of our connectedness to ourselves, to each other, to our bodies, to our physical earth, and to the universe. There is nothing else.

We live our lives as if our physical bodies make us separate and alone. We are not separate from each other in learning how best to live physically while fulfilling our spiritual purpose. This is our human commonality - our relationship with our bodies and ourselves.

Your body enables you to taste the food you love, hum a tune, see the beauty of a smile, and hear the music. Your body enables you to step across the room, dream while you sleep, and hug those you love.

Your body is not your enemy; it hasn't sabotaged your pleasure. It doesn't deserve your hate. You pour toxic poisonous food into it and your body works endlessly to clean it out.

And to heal. And when you do it again, your body starts the whole process over.

Your body never says to you, "I hate what you're feeding me, I hate you." Instead, your body says, "I will make energy from what you have given me. I will move you closer to whatever you desire with the energy I make. I will gulp bad air and poisonous food and I will sit in one position even though it causes me pain, if that is what you want me to do. I am here to serve you. I am your best and oldest friend in this lifetime. I know you when you are tired, and sad, and when you hate me, I will still take what you give me and make energy for you. I love you. I forgive you, I'm sorry if what I do is not enough. Thank you for being one with me."

This is the essence of Ho'oponopono Healing, an ancient tribal Hawaiian method of negotiating with the enemy. By looking inside your own heart, you negotiated with the enemy who wanted to destroy you. You could not do anything about the other person. You could only change how you felt. And by changing how you felt about the enemy, they changed how they behaved toward you.

Obese people have become enemies to their bodies. They view their bodies as traitors, ugly horrible things that have failed them.

Try this exercise with your body. Talk to your body with these sentences, doing so is the beginning of learning to love this physical essence that is working so hard for you, even though you may hate and mistreat it.

Ho'oponopono Healing Exercise

(for you and your body)

I'm sorry

I'm sorry that I mistreat you by pouring junk food in you.

I'm sorry that I do not understand your messages.

I love

I love myself for learning how to be kind to you.

I love you for sticking with me while I learn.

I forgive

I forgive myself for all the harm I have done to you and for not knowing any better.

I forgive you for being less than perfect.

Thank you

I thank myself for trying to heal you.

Thank you for trying to keep going.

Section Three

Life Begins Tomorrow, I'll Start When I'm Thin
Sex And Love: They Fixed Me Up With The Fat Kid
Black Is My Favorite Color: The Price Tag Of Shame

Chapter
13

Life Begins Tomorrow, I'll Start When I'm Thin

Some people mark the cycles of their lives by their life events: birthdays, graduations, marriages, births, and deaths. Others mark their lives in terms of years: this age, that age, when I was a teenager, when I turned 40. Still others number their days according to stages of life: elementary school, high school, college, work, family, and illness.

I mark my life by how many pounds I weighed. And by how many pounds overweight that was for me.

I mark my life by how many events I missed. Or by the ones I attended and wished I hadn't.

I avoided swim parties or volleyball games or learning to ski. I told people I wasn't interested in weddings, and proms, and dates and parties.

I remember how much I weighed in every grade, at every graduation, and at every season. Until at some point, I weighed the same and stopped weighing myself.

I lied on every driver's license about my weight. As if the picture didn't show the truth.

I stayed home on nice days rather than go to amusement parks and show my arms.

I avoided dates and sexual activity because I was embarrassed about how I looked.

I delayed and delayed my wedding waiting for thinness. When my husband told me he loved me, I did not believe it was possible.

These are not pleasant memories to recall. I do not write them with pride or pleasure.

I became an observer to other people's lives, rather than a participant in my own.

I was a friend, I could listen. I was just not an attendee.

I missed my childhood. I missed my teen years. I missed my young adulthood. I stayed home with my self-image and my cookies.

On those rare occasions where I showed up, and someone would compliment me, "nice dress… your hair looks good… I like your makeup", I responded, "No. It's old, it's ugly, it's nothing."

I don't look nice. I'm not pretty. I don't deserve your compliment.

I cannot tolerate you telling me my physical body has beauty because I know that I am disgusting and it does not.

My truth of experience and feeling is stronger than your truth of observation. Inside me, I feel I am without beauty.

I am not telling you this so you will feel sorry for me or for you. I tell you this because it is what we do as human beings with less than perfect bodies. Whether it's weight, or hair, or skin, or height or some other physical attribute. Whether it's how we look, or speak or dress. We put our lives on hold because tomorrow will be better. Life will be better when I'm thin. Or maybe just after I eat.

I don't think this is just human behavior. This morning my male Newfoundland dog eagerly ran outside to play fetch before breakfast. My female Newfie (the one with the weight problem) sat alone inside waiting for breakfast and watching us through the window. No amount of cajoling and open doors could get her to get up and come out before she ate. The call in her heart at that moment was for food. Not fun.

As a child, I remember eating endless cookies at other people's homes. What did their mothers say when they saw that?

After a while, I was embarrassed to eat in front of people. I never ate in front of friends. One day, in my 20's at a friend's house with a few other people, I politely declined his offering of food, "Oh, that's right", he said, "you're a secret eater".

Outed - with one sentence by a guy I hardly knew. Just a statement of fact. Not said with malice, just stated like you would acknowledge a person's peanut allergy. You're a secret eater. You're allergic to eating in public.

It was that obvious.

My substitution was work and fantasy, and work-fantasy. Sometimes I would imagine the future when I was thin, and gorgeous and how amazed people would be when they saw me. Sometimes I would simply work and use that as an excuse for not living. I cannot be there to celebrate because I am enslaved.

The reality was that I was only enslaved to my embarrassment, not to any overly demanding boss or parent.

It was almost always an excuse to avoid being with others, to avoid celebrating the fullness and happiness of their lives and having nothing to offer up in return. How often can you talk about work when other people talk about dates, and families and trips? How often can you talk about your dogs when other people talk about their kids?

I missed the excitement, the exhilaration, the joy, the contentment, the beauty of all of those occasions. I traded a chance at fulfillment for an hour or two of self-imposed suffering because I could not bear to bring my obese body to an event. I cannot get those moments back, but I do not have to continue the pattern.

To all of you, and to myself, I tell you what Ram Dass said forty years ago: **Be here now.**

Here is where you are now. This is who you are now. One of the reasons you are reading this is because you do not feel the way you look.

Bring your essential self - your soul, your very being - to every place, and every event and every moment. Forget your body. It changes everyday.

And to all of my friends, and family, and coworkers, and colleagues, and classmates and strangers, forgive me for the moments I missed, I'm sorry for the moments I missed, thank you for the invitations and the inclusions. I love you for thinking of me, I think of you, too.

I met my husband on the Internet. We began by conversing. For me, it bypassed the issue of how I thought I looked, and allowed me to present my authentic self.

Recently, I read a wonderful story about a woman who lost many hundreds of pounds and appeared on *Oprah*. She never left her apartment. She had no friends. Until she found the Internet. There she began to converse about interesting topics with like-minded people. For the first time in many years, she started to form friendships. She began to experience the oneness of relating to others. She used this as a tool to reshape her life and her body.

I am often asked in my role as a psychiatrist whether real friendships can be formed online. The answer is yes. At some point, I recommend the friendships move offline to telephone, if not in-person, to provide spontaneity that does not exist when typing.

If you are housebound, if you are unable, or uncomfortable or unwilling to go out, begin by socializing with like-minded people on the Internet. (Yes, you do have to be cautious; most Internet Service Providers (ISP's) have information on staying safe.)

Allow your real self to emerge online. Then bring your real self to life events in-person.

Chapter
14

Sex And Love: They Fixed Me Up With The Fat Kid

I kept waiting to write this chapter thinking there would be many memories, they would be painful but this would be easy to write.

I was wrong.

It was not painful.

It was impossible.

As I struggled to remember, every seam on my pants began to squeeze. My comfortable clothes started to cling and my skin screamed for the chafing to stop. A few hours ago I had raced up and down the hallway at work, laughing and gesturing freely. Now, suddenly, I was completely locked up in skin that was too tight for my body. I didn't fit right.

My body was remembering what my mind could not.

Meanwhile, I couldn't remember many incidents, just a few, and they all seemed the same - uncomfortable, awkward, and ill fitting. And my brain was begging me to please forget, just as my pants were begging me to please change into clothes that fit.

This is a chapter on sex and I couldn't remember anything that felt sexual. What I remember is how my clothes didn't fit, my body didn't fit, and my sense of self didn't fit.

Obese children mature sooner. I was 9 years old when I got my period. I wasn't the first in my class; there was a girl who looked 15 and had to change for swimming with the camp counselors. I was the second. And I was young enough that I had needed help from my mother managing the hygiene. She used to shave me under the arms because I was too young to hold a razor.

I was 11 years old when I went to summer camp in the Blue Ridge Mountains. The location was beautiful, but I'd never been away from home, and none of my friends were with me. I was miserable. It didn't help that there were "socials" every Saturday night that involved dancing with boys. Just the thought of it made me tongue-tied and anxious. The other girls - skinny, lithe, lively girls – danced with cute grinning boys. They conspired to fix me up with the lone fat boy, who was the same age. It was obvious to them that we belonged together. It wasn't cruelty, it was symmetry. The male fat kid. My clone.

I didn't see his inner beauty. I saw the other fat, awkward kid who was as embarrassed as I was.

When I went to a different camp a year later, a grown-up male cook who worked there smiled at me. He tried to kiss me and I ran away. I never told anyone – it was gross, and weird, and didn't feel good and I knew it.

When there were parties, I was invited, but no boy would dance with me. There I was with my fancy too-tight-feeling chubby dress, in painful low heels with my thighs chafing together in stockings. I hung out with the punch bowl and the moms. Always helpful, I was great at clean-up.

My underwear resembled "garments". In the seventh grade, I played violin in the orchestra. During a rehearsal, my bra strap popped with a resounding snap breaking a moment of silence. The high school boys started laughing. I tried to deny my elastic failure, but it was useless. The weight of my breasts had the last sound.

I remember looking at an obese teacher with an obese wife and wondering how they "did" it. Their stomachs would get in the way, I thought.

When I look back at pictures of myself as a teenager, I see a very beautiful girl. I never felt that, even with my best makeup and outfit. I felt fat. And ugly. And embarrassed. And those feelings tainted every moment of my life growing up from the time my weight problem began, sometime in elementary school.

I was the girl that was every boy's friend. Boys asked to copy my homework regularly. I was a senior in high school in the spring (during mating season), and one of the nicer cuter boys in my class put his arm around me tenderly in a moment of friendship and said, "You're the only girl that I could be naked with all night long and not have sex".

Thank you. I will do my best to continue being as asexual as possible. Despite my inner longings. Despite my raging hormones. Despite my beating heart. I will do my best to wear tents and ignore the chafing between my legs.

Then there was the other group of boys. The teenage versions of the camp cook. Those that assumed that fat girls put out. That a fat girl would be darn lucky to have this boy even touch her. That it doesn't matter if you make fun of her because she's subhuman anyway.

There is a rhythm of learning sexuality. First, you learn to think and feel, then look, then talk, then play. Hormones are meant to come later, after a child has a chance to practice a few social skills. Like tag and softball. Like giggling and blushing. Like dreaming and playing. Touch comes much later.

Obesity in young girls and boys changes that natural timeline. Suddenly, a child with no social preparation is a raging hormonal mess. A 9 year-old with an adult body. Who shouldn't be staying up past 9:30. Who cannot handle the sensations and doesn't know what they mean. The weight becomes a barrier to love for both genders, rendering children less attractive, less confident, and less interested in themselves and others. Moving touch to occurring either too early on the timeline or never at all.

Eventually, if the person weighs enough, they lose their sex drive. At any age.

I threw myself into work for 20 years. When I finally met a man I loved and who loved me, I struggled to believe that he found me attractive. It wasn't the truth I had known for most of my life.

I had to start from the beginning. As an adult, I had to learn how to be a teenager. How to talk, how to caress, how to romance, how to giggle. How to explore. How to respond. How to play. This wasn't about how to have sex. This was about how to be physically and emotionally loved in a joyful sexual way.

Sometimes patients in my office need to talk about sex - the 'hows and the whys' and the 'why can't I's'. The patients often seem surprised to hear a fat psychiatrist talk about sex.

Which allows me to revisit my lessons in endearing and strange ways.

A 30-something woman came in about a year after successful bariatric surgery, complaining of an increase in alcohol consumption every night. She was happy with her weight loss, had a good marriage and supportive husband, was satisfied with her job, and did not have serious financial or parenting issues. Both of her parents were alive and well.

Her only stressor was that she did not want her husband to touch her.

Aha! screams the novice therapist. She's been abused!

But the patient had not been abused, and had previously enjoyed sex with her husband very much, despite being 100 pounds heavier. He was in love with her no matter her size, and had not changed his lovemaking habits at all. Nothing seemed different, and yet, she had to drink two drinks every night in case he wanted to have sex. The strange part of this, for her, was that she wanted to have sex, too. But she couldn't stand it now.

Being obese changes the way sex feels - and losing weight changes it again. This is not just about being in the mood, although being in the mood certainly will help.

Excess weight in the abdomen compresses female sexual organs, functionally causing the vagina to feel shorter. Both obesity and diabetes decrease nerve sensation in the genital areas; as a result, both women and men may need more manual stimulation in order to reach orgasm.

When women lose weight, they feel as if they have more vaginal surface area or improved sensation, and the amount of pressure previously required to stimulate may now seem painful. Changing from a woman on the bottom to woman on the top position can alleviate some of this change.

Obese men often have retracted penises due to abdominal fat. This may be mistaken as a hernia or may mask a hernia. Losing weight changes penile length by shrinking the abdominal fold. Functionally, the male penis seems longer.

Experimenting with changes in position, techniques and sexual aids can assist someone who has lost or gained a significant amount of weight feel comfortable during sex.

To be comfortable and sexual requires concentration. And the easiest place and way to concentrate is to feel where the energy is growing:

Sometimes in your heart when you are being loved.

Sometimes in your body when you are touching and being touched.

Sometimes in your brain when you are joining.

Your mind, your body and your spirit are all sexual organs.

You have a sex life regardless of your size.

Chapter
15

Black Is My Favorite Color: The Price Tag of Shame

Appearance is our introduction. How we look is what other people see when they meet us.

Our outer appearance is also a reflection of how we feel within. If I am uncomfortable with how I look, I am handing out the message that I am uncomfortable with how I feel about myself. And inviting you to feel the same way about me.

What does it feel like to love your body? I wonder.

What does it feel like to be dressed in sleek clothing that fits no matter how you move?

What does it feel like to be somewhere warm and sunny and let your arms and legs show and have tight skin and strong muscles and a healthy tan?

What does it feel like to know that you look great even when you're walking around with no makeup and flip-flops?

Sounds silly, doesn't it.

It's the sound of a fat teenaged girl. It's the sound of a fat young woman. It's the sound of a middle-aged fat woman. The sound is much softer than when I was young, but if I listen in the changing room with the mirrors, I hear it.

It is the sound of obesity looking in the mirror.

By the time I was in the second grade, I was obese. I remember measuring my size against other little girls my age while I was in advanced beginners swimming and ballet classes. We have an innate recognition of "cute", and I knew those girls had it. I wanted nothing more than to be one of them.

If I couldn't look like them, then maybe I could be athletic like the other not so cute but skinny girls around me. It wasn't to be. No matter how hard I tried, I couldn't run fast, throw hard, or move fast. Not cute and not quick.

I didn't fit in girls sizes; I didn't fit in junior sizes; I didn't fit in women sizes.

There was a little clothing area with chubby girl clothes in a dingy corner of the local department store basement between the bathroom and the elevator. There wasn't much to choose from; the few clothes they had were dowdy and old-looking, as if fat kids should dress like their grandmothers. My mother would do her best to find me a "shift" that was a pretty color. That provided some small amount of optical illusion so I didn't look as big as I was.

No horizontal stripes or loud prints. No sleeveless. No tuck-ins or wide belts.

I always loved that carnival mirror that made you look really tall and thin. For a minute or two I had the fantasy of normal weight.

The doctor wrote down "morbid obesity" in my chart. I was mortified. I looked it up. It meant I was going to die from being fat. I was 12.

I remember going to a swim party as a young teen and swimming in shorts and a t-shirt. I remember being dressed in chubby girl clothes at a dance, having worked very hard to put that outfit and my hair and my first lip gloss together, and not being asked to dance.

I remember being on the balance beam in high school and seeing a teacher's face turn from a hearty smile to a mask of shock as he walked by and waved, never having seen me in my gym uniform.

I remember my much older cousin having a friend who was morbidly obese. I remember being horrified at the size of her thighs – they seemed as wide as sidewalks. I remember thinking I'll never be like that. I am. I think I am.

I developed the perfect wardrobe. Black. Black jackets. Black pants. Black shoes. Maybe a little color in my shirt. How many pounds could I hide wearing a boxy black jacket. 10? 20? I was 150 pounds overweight – what's 10 pounds going to do?

It's going to help me feel a tiny bit less embarrassed about my size. It's going to give me the illusion that no one notices. It's going to hide the telltale stain down the front of my shirt. Evidence. The fat girl eats and she's a slob.

One day my dear aunt and I were standing as adults in her kitchen discussing clothes. "You wouldn't wear that" she said, "You like those big jackets that hide your weight." She was right, she was factual. And I was outed once again, and embarrassed. Somebody noticed.

I tried the being "big and happy" way of thinking. Big and beautiful. Maybe there are people out there who actually feel that way, I wasn't one of them. I do occasionally meet someone who feels that big is normal for them, their family, their culture. But they are not happy about it. I wasn't happy about it, I didn't love my body. I hated that clothes didn't fit, I had difficulty moving, I felt pain and low energy, people looked away from me. I hated that the person in the mirror did not seem to be the same person in my mind.

I remember being embarrassed that Mama Cass choked to death. She didn't choke actually, she had a heart attack, but I never knew that until recently. I was ashamed that John Belushi and John Candy and Chris Farley died of excesses. I cringed when I saw Jackie Gleason and Dom DeLuise and Luciano Pavarotti and Nell Carter. I hated that Marlon Brando and Elvis became obese. I felt so sad that Jerry Garcia died too soon. I shook my head in dismay when Kirstie Alley went on a crash diet with the tabloids on her heels. I didn't understand how Christina Onassis could have all that money and still grapple with her weight. Oprah's and Roseanne's and Aretha's weight struggles hurt, I feel pain, I love them and I want them to be well. I could not write this book without their very public struggle.

These days I'm doing better with my health and weight, but still wearing black. It is my comfort zone. Flowered pants make me intensely curious. Who wears those?

I went to exercise class not too long ago, a class I enjoy that actually feels like fun. A talkative older lady told me to keep up the good work in class, I was "a pretty girl" and it was good for me. When I told her that I had just lost 40 pounds, she recoiled and said "how could you let yourself get that way??!"

My comfort with my appearance is a deeply personal and now deeply spiritual experience of my physical body that is held within me. It is essential, it is historical, it is influenced, it is environmental. It is the truth of *HOW I FEEL*, not how I look.

Now if I could just convince everyone else.

Section Four

If You Know So Much, Why Are You Still Fat?
I'm Only Allowed Ten Grapes: Is The Medical Community
Helping Or Hurting?
Where Do I Begin?
The Last Unanswered Prejudice: You Are Not Alone

Chapter
16

If You Know So Much, Why Are You Still Fat?

> *"The Torah speaks of four types of children:*
> *one who is wise, one who is rebellious,*
> *one who is simple, and one who does not know how*
> *to ask."*
>
> — *Passover Haggadah*

This section of the book is for healthcare providers working with obese patients. Maybe they will read this. Maybe they will not. Maybe you will be the one to educate your healthcare provider on how best to work with you and your weight. Unfortunately, most healthcare providers do not know what works best for obesity. They may not know what works best for you individually, either. It is YOUR responsibility to yourself to be your own advocate, and be your own spokesperson.

I'm going to teach you how to talk to your doctor, your nutritionist, and your therapist about your weight.

Once, I was teaching a seminar for a team of bariatric surgery providers. We had reviewed emotional connections, emotional eating, addiction, brain chemistry, plus how best to convey a sense of purpose and hope to a very defeated population. I thought, as did my colleague next to me, that I had done a pretty good job of explaining the pitfalls of treating patients with lifelong obesity, and offered some decent suggestions on helping them successfully navigate the bariatric surgery process.

When I work with obese patients and we discuss weight, or when I work with addicted patients and we discuss addiction, it's natural for me to motion to my body and tell them "it's not like I know all the answers; I'm still searching, too". I had done this several times during the seminar, lightly touching on my self-awareness without giving too many details. I was, and still am, largely a grief, stress/anxiety and energy eater. I eat too many sweets and carbohydrates, and I exercise too little. I work too much, and leave too little time to cool down my body and my brain between challenges. (At that time, I did not understand the role that food intolerances played in my addiction.)

One of the bariatric providers looked like she had a question, but was having difficulty asking. Always the psychiatrist, I encouraged her to simply ask, there isn't a stupid question. "Okay", she said, "well, if you know so much, why are you still fat?"

It was not the first time anyone has stated the obvious, but usually I am the one who controls the timing. I was unprepared for the emotional shock that reverberated through me.

The question was obvious. Good for her for having the courage to ask. The delivery, on the other hand…not so good.

Retrospectively, I have her to thank for this book. Why didn't anyone else ask that question? Why was I so offended when someone finally did?

Without that very public challenge, I could have continued to fool myself *that no one would notice*.

I think back about my health care providers, about myself as a health care provider, and about the stories of health care providers I've heard over the years. They range from too much compassion, to ignoring the problem, to complete hostility and dislike for the obese patient.

I remember being in the operating room when a surgeon called an anesthetized obese woman a "beached whale".

I remember having a doctor tell me (at my very middle weight, nowhere near my heaviest) that I was "packing a lot of weight around that middle".

I have routinely encountered doctors who look right past my weight and complain about obese patients. Do they see me as an obese patient? Or do they see me as a physician qualified to discuss obesity? And if they do see me as qualified, how do they explain the discrepancy between what they see and how I look?

Most doctors are not cruel or hostile to fat people, they are simply at a loss for doctor-like words. When they reach into their toolbox of healthy conversations, the one on losing weight is scratched and worn-out. Most doctors no longer even try to muster the enormous amount of energy needed to coach someone through weight loss.

They are at a loss.

You can help the doctors.

They need you to remind them that your life is worth saving.

They need you to remind them that you may be difficult, but you are not hopeless.

They need you to remind them that all their training really can help you, if they will just be patient and not give up.

For the doctor who is wise, talk from the heart, "Doctor, I do not want to live like this, can you help me?" Tell them that you are afraid. Ask him where do you start. Ask him for reassurance that he will not abandon you if you fail.

For the doctor who is hostile, talk from the brain, "Doctor, I know I have not listened to your advice, I know how frustrated you are with me. Will you help me try again?" Show her your frailty, and let her remember your humanness.

For the doctor who is simple, talk from the gut. No excuses, no fancy talk, no reasons why. "Doctor, I don't know how I will do, but I promise I will try."

And for the doctor who does not know how to ask, talk from your soul, "Doctor, please do not overlook my weight. I have struggled for years and I have failed often. This is my story, but I would like to try again. I will do what you tell me to do, I will do the best I can do, and I will return as often as you say is necessary."

Your healthcare is a partnership between you and your healthcare providers. We are neither your enemies, nor your saviors. We are simply people. We have worked many hard years to give you the benefit of our education and experience. We do not know everything. This epidemic of obesity has us stumped. But even when we do not know the answers or have all the tools, we have taken an oath to do the best we can to help you. Do not forsake that offer.

Chapter

17

I'm Only Allowed Ten Grapes: Is the Medical Community Helping or Hurting?

A frustrated internist referred a middle-aged woman with Type 2 Diabetes to me. She weighed well over 400 pounds and had out of control blood sugars. Her weight was steadily increasing. She swore up and down to the doctor and the nurses that she took her medicine and followed the diabetes-eating plan. An endocrinologist had tested her for additional metabolic abnormalities, but found nothing unexpected. No "slow metabolism" problem we all wish we had.

She was talkative and entertaining, a frequent depression mask that obese patients use in order to be liked and accepted.

After awhile, we came to the topic of her blood sugars and her weight. "What are you eating that could be causing a problem here?" I asked.

"Nothing bad", came the usual 'I-don't-want-to-get-yelled-at-by-the-doctor' answer.

"I'm not here to judge you, I just want to see if there are some changes we can make in your medications or your lifestyle that will be easy for you."

It turned out that every night she ate cookies, and candy and ice cream in large quantities. "I can't stay away from it", she said, the sure-fire sign of a brain searching for more dopamine and serotonin, and a body that can't transport sugar from the bloodstream inside a cell.

Well, okay, let's analyze this. It turned out that this particular patient had a sugar addiction in response to depression, anxiety and fear of being alone. Her sugar mechanism was faulty due to her diabetic insulin resistance. This meant that, even though her blood sugar was 300, there were no working transporters to carry that sugar into the cell where it was needed. Inside the cell, her energy-producing mitochondria were starving and screaming to her brain to bring them more sugar!

We start in the beginning in cases like this. The first goal is to stop the sugar binging. I use medications and some minor dietary changes to start. Refined sugar is easy to replace – there are many substitutes. We started with the most obvious. "How about fruit? Do you like fruit?" I asked, thinking that perhaps half of the refined sugar could be replaced by something healthier.

Another similar story… the other day we were walking our dogs on a beautiful early summer day in Northeast Ohio, where weather is always a topic. We shared weather admiration with an older neighbor finishing up her afternoon stroll. Her walk, it turns out, was unplanned, a reaction to feeling "horrible anxiety" inside.

"I knew I'd feel better if I took a little walk."

"Maybe you can sit outside a little and soak up some more Vitamin D and your beautiful flowers?", I said, motioning at a yard filled with flowers and scent and color.

"No, I can't", she said, "I'm on medication that reacts with the sun. I have to stay in."

"I love fruit! Grapes! I love grapes!"

"Could you buy some grapes and eat those every night first? It might cost a little more, but you wouldn't be buying as much cookies and candy, so it would probably even out financially."

"I can't", she said. "I'm not allowed."

"Why?" I wondered aloud, "Are you allergic?"

"Oh no", she replied. "I'm not allergic to grapes. They told me I'm only allowed to have ten grapes at a time. That's one serving."

WHAT ARE WE DOING????

Is the medical establishment hurting or helping patients lose weight?

We are prescribing medications that cause weight gain, fatigue, loss of sex drive, increase in appetite, memory loss, and anxiety and restlessness.

We lowered your cholesterol, but you can't get off the couch and go for a walk.

We lowered your blood sugar, but you gained weight.

We treated your depression, but you can't stop eating sweets and now you're on the verge of diabetes.

We treated your blood pressure but now your potassium is dangerously low and you're having muscle spasms.

You become addicted to pain killers, sedatives, sleeping pills, nerve pills, and uppers and diet pills so that you think, sleep, relax, and work and not overeat.

To treat the side effects of obesity, we are prescribing medications that cause more side effects, including more obesity. *The very side effects that might act as a deterrent to eating foods that are causing weight gain.*

If the high fat, spicy meal gives you heartburn, you might not eat it anymore. But if we give you a pill to take away the heartburn, you can eat all you want. Even if that meal blocks your absorption of energy-producing vitamin B12.

Your body may stop digesting dairy products when you reach adulthood. That's because the purpose of milk is to rapidly grow a 50-pound calf into a 600-pound heifer. It is meant to grow your body. When you are fully grown, your body starts to reject milk. But don't fear, we can treat all of those digestive symptoms so you can eat unlimited dairy products and continue your body growth.

We can effectively silence your body's complaints about what you eat. We can override your body's normal mechanisms so that your entire metabolism is out of balance, but you're able to eat to your heart's content.

We will reimburse all of these medications if you are insured. We will put the old ones on sale if you are not. But you're on your own with fresh fruit and gym memberships.

When the lady who was binging on cookies and candy every night told me about the grapes, I made her a deal. I gave her special doctor-permission to eat all the fruit she wanted for the next 30 days. She could also eat cookies or candy if she desired; the only rule was she had to have her fill of fruit first, she had to eat two popsicles first before ice cream, and she had to drink 2 to 3 cups of green tea and eat 2 to 4 ounces of dark chocolate everyday.

And she had to silently bless the food she ate and the body she fed every time she ate.

She lost 20 pounds that month. Her blood sugar dropped below 200 for the first time in months. She came back to my office, smiling broadly, "This is a great diet."

I hope the medical system will change. I hope insurers will begin to reimburse for foods, and treatments and supplements that heal, and keep us whole and healthy. I hope that our places of work will become institutions of robust activity and well-being. I hope that the advice doctors dispense to people who are obese becomes sensible and easy to follow.

In the meantime, there are changes you can make that will help your body heal. In the next chapter, I will give you a place to begin.

No boot camp. No starvation. No more stress.

Just a moment-to-moment living, breathing affirmation that your life is valuable and your body is worth saving.

You are not a disease. Your body may have a disease, but that is not who you are. In medical school we were carefully taught never to talk about a person by their illness – they were not "the Gall Bladder in Room 26"; they were Mrs. Jones with gallstones. Yet we call people "diabetic". Not a person with diabetes – we are describing human beings as diseases, particularly diseases of obesity.

We would never refer to someone as a "canceric" or a "heart attackic". Do not call yourself a disease any longer and correct the providers who may not know any better. Obesity is a label of your body, not the state of your soul.

Chapter

18

Where Do I Begin?

Begin at the beginning. Begin by practicing loving kindness toward yourself and your body. If you have read this far, then you know that I do not support adding stress to your life, either mentally or physically. I do support getting all the help you need to live the life you desire.

Here are the first steps. Make sure they are baby steps so you do not become overwhelmed or discouraged. Change things slowly and stay within your comfort zone. Ask your body for permission for each change, and thank it for helping you with this transition. Your body will thank you back by healing.

1. Slowly detoxify your body.

Start easily, not with a drastic colon cleanse that will land you in the Emergency Room. Start by improving the quality of the food you eat. One of the reasons we binge is that there are not enough satisfying nutrients and flavors in poor quality food, and we want more. Don't fill your body with toxic chemicals that are worsening your depression and disrupting your sleep and memory and sex life. Read labels – if you cannot pronounce the name of an ingredient, and you cannot picture what it looks like, *it isn't food. It's POISON.*

Look up the foods that are healthy for you, and try eating one everyday. After awhile, try to eat two of them. This is a meal plan of adding, not subtracting.

DO NOT DENY yourself any foods, unless you are detoxifying a specific medical condition, such as allergy or heavy metal poisoning. Denying foods is a sure set-up for a binge. Better to work with the cravings by anticipating that they will occur daily, and plan ahead.

Beware of diets that TELL YOU what you should be eating. I was never sicker than when I was on a vegan diet. My chest pain went away, I lost weight, but it turned out I was allergic to most of the protein sources I was eating. It works great for some, not so great for others. Learn to LISTEN to your body's signals.

Your body has essential wisdom. It tells you what chemical it needs to produce a balance in your brain. Your job is to supply your body with the highest quality ingredients available.

If you improve the quality of your food, the quantity you eat will diminish naturally. Not instantly. Naturally. The price of your food when you are eating less, is probably the same.

Food and emotions work in two directions. Unhealthy foods can cause unwanted emotions. Unwanted emotions cause cravings for specific foods.

Put together a list of foods that affect your brain chemistry and improve your mood, and then stock up on them. Eat them daily. Mark Hyman, M.D. has a great program called "The UltraMind Solution" that links different feelings with different foods. Imagine if you can eat away your anxiety by adding turkey. (It works for me!)

If you are craving sugar, first eat fresh fruit. At least get a vitamin or two with your sweetness! Hopefully, you will eat fewer cookies if they are dessert to the fruit. For ice cream cravings, eat two popsicles BEFORE you eat the ice cream.

Salty, crunchy food cravings are often the result of anger and frustration. Move away from table salt toward sea salt. Add hot and spicy to your craving food – eat spicy dips such as salsa or guacamole, put Tabasco or peppers on your meal.

CRAVINGS

The reason you are eating such large quantities of cheap chocolate is because there is SO LITTLE chocolate in each candy bar. If your body wants serotonin and magnesium, then give it some.

For chocolate cravings, eat two bananas, several cups of green tea and 2 to 4 ounces of very dark chocolate (70% or more) every day. EVERY DAY. After awhile, the cravings will go away.

Make it your habit to use healthy fats, such as olive oil and sesame oil. Learn to use spices to add flavor. Keep a supply of cooked food in your refrigerator that is the basis for your meal – I keep a fresh supply of cooked chicken, guacamole and salsa, cut up vegetables, soup, fruit, 85% dark chocolate and popsicles. I always have cooked rice or sweet potatoes available. When I want or need to eat in a hurry, the food is there.

Eat the real thing. If you want corn, eat corn, not syrup. Seek the real comfort. Ice cream is not a hug. It simply makes you forget you needed one.

Do not neglect protein in favor of carbohydrates because you are counting calories or quantities. You cannot run your body without protein. Your skin will not heal, you cannot think, you will not have energy or desire sex.

Beware of "health food". The ingredients in "baked" chips may be much more toxic than the old-fashioned kind. Remember, if you cannot pronounce it, and you cannot picture it, it's not food - it's POISON.

2. Interrupt those automatic negative thoughts. Constantly.

In the beginning, do not try to substitute happy affirmations – they will not ring true with all that pain in your soul. Recognize that some of what you are thinking is exaggerated and maybe even irrational. Some of what you are thinking can be reversed. The simple act of recognizing, "Oh here I go again" will stop the thought. In the beginning, you might have to interrupt yourself 1,000 times an hour. Like all habits, automatic negative thinking can be overcome.

In time, you will begin to believe those affirmations and they will help interrupt the negative thoughts.

Limit your exposure to negative thought makers such as violence, news stories, AND heated arguments. They will always make you feel worse. Walk away. Change the station. Open the drapes. I am not saying do not be informed. I am saying do not suffer someone else's misfortune. You cannot take on their pain because PAIN IS NOT TRANSFERABLE. Watching someone whose home was destroyed in a disaster and feeling badly does not rebuild their home or help them. Say a prayer, send an email, knit a sweater, or make your own home safer and your own life better. Make something good come out of something bad. It is how we heal ourselves and the world.

3. Move

Even if it's just your arms. Breathe as deeply as you can. Stretch your arms out. Feel your heart beating. Wiggle your fingers. Your body is alive and wants to be active. Even a little motion will increase your energy. GET SOME FRESH AIR.

I don't "workout". I move, I walk, I have fun. My goal is to ski again and hike beautiful high mountains. I like the way my back feels when I stretch and do certain exercises. I like the way my arms feel when I lift (not-too-heavy) weights.

4. Change it up.

Change anything you can. Change chairs, desserts, your route at work, what you eat. Any change will help. Change will evoke a natural sense of curiosity. Even if you change to something you do not like, you will have made your day more interesting.

5. Surround yourself with beauty and spirit.

I'm not talking about anything expensive. I'm talking about music that brings you joy, walking past a flower garden that smells wonderful, saying a prayer or noticing the sky. There is another truth out there besides the broken record in your mind. Take time for yourself. Yes, I know you work full-time, and go to school full-time and are raising a family as a single parent. But you are no good to anyone, including yourself, unless you can quiet your mind and reconnect with your heart. Close the bathroom door and spend an extra 10 minutes reading a meditation or just enjoying the quiet. Yes, the bathroom.

6. Do something for someone else.

Yes you are having a hard time. Someone else has it worse. I can guarantee that. And someone else will benefit from your kindness and caring, even if it means simply saying hello to them instead of rushing past with unseeing eyes. Hold the door for someone. Let them in your lane.

7. Take supplements

Yes, I recommend supplements. If you have depression, take 3-omega fatty acids 1,000 mg twice daily. This is the "oil and lube" for your brain. Take a multivitamin AND mineral pill, and get your Vitamin D level checked unless you live at the equator or play golf in the sun everyday. There are many other supplements available. Talk to your doctor or visit reliable websites listed in the Resources section of this book.

8. Relax Your Mind.

I need assisted meditations and guided imageries to relax and also to fall asleep. If I try to quiet my mind without headphones, I hear every little sound and think of every little task. The silly ocean waves and wind chimes help me tune everything else out. If you have trouble sleeping as a result of depression, or are experiencing early morning or mid-sleep cycle awakening, use the time to do a guided imagery or meditation.

If you cannot sleep, stay away from the computer. The computer acts as a stimulant in your brain – it's speed. It awakens multiple areas of activity simultaneously. That is why you can sit down to play a game on the computer and three hours later you're not tired.

Okay, so now you know what to do. A little change in food, a little movement, a little meditation, a little more sleep…

A little more enjoyment.

A little more peace.

A lot more health.

You can do this; I know that because I did it. And everyday I am grateful.

Chapter
19

The Last Unanswered
Prejudice: You Are Not Alone

Obesity is the last unanswered prejudice. It is acceptable in society to ignore, demean, degrade, to be openly hostile toward, and to generally overlook obese individuals.

As an adult:

I have seen people look away from my smile when I pass them, rather than make eye contact.

I have had sales people walk past me with no interest in promoting their product, even though I have a credit card and a readiness to buy.

When I was a surgical resident, my surgeon boss-of-the-month instructed me to walk up twenty-two flights of stairs in the hospital right then-and-there to get in shape. In all fairness, the attending surgeon and the chief resident surgeon (both committed to working out and competing with each other) went up those steps, too. Again, in all fairness, I didn't have the nerve to say, "No, I can't or I don't want to."

A group of men screamed insults at me from a passing car while I rode a bicycle. I was not allowed to rent a scooter at a resort.

A deliveryman told me to unload my own boxes from a delivery truck because I was obviously big enough to handle them.

I was called names at a professional meeting with sexual references about my weight, when my colleagues and I went to a restaurant for dinner. (I was so shocked, I couldn't respond).

I had a *faculty psychiatrist* verbally attack me in front of peers and later admit he hated fat people.

I was not provocative or asking for confrontation in any of those circumstances. I was simply existing within a social or professional structure, such as work or public recreation or dining out. I was shopping, riding a bicycle, presenting a report, socializing with coworkers.

I can't even begin to report the childhood incidences. There are so many, and I have effectively blocked most of them from conscious memory.

Obese people are passed over for jobs and denied promotions.

Obese people are denied entrance to schools and associations.

Obese people are scorned, openly derided.

Obese people are the subject of jokes and hostility in the media.

Obese people receive less aggressive medical care.

Obese people are paid less for the same work.

Obese people receive worse customer service in stores and may pay more for the same products.

Obese children receive less education and lower grades than others, despite the same IQ .

Obese parents are denied adoptions.

Obese people are perceived as sloppy, lazy and "repulsive" by medical professionals who claim to *be trained in obesity*; causing obese people to avoid medical care.

I can hear the pundits on this one already, "The obese people deserve it, they did it to themselves, they are responsible for what they put in their mouths. They are weak, they are making excuses, they are pathetic, they are lazy."

This is not a chapter about whether or not we contribute to our own obesity. Of course we do. This is a chapter about whether we are mistreated by others because of our obesity.

This chapter is about the color of your skin.

This chapter is about the religion you practice.

This chapter is about your country or ethnic group of origin.

This chapter is about your gender.

This chapter is about your height.

This chapter is about your sexual preference.

This chapter is about your politics.

This chapter is about being hated for who you seem to be. By someone who doesn't know who you are.

This chapter is about being judged.

This chapter is about how we have the capacity to hate each other because of insignificant minor differences. Rather than see potential, beauty, creativity, and humor, we all, at times, choose to see something in someone else that enables us to feel superior. If I say you are fat and stupid, it implies I am thin and smart.

I don't know what advice to give when you are discriminated against or taunted or violated because of your weight. It required years of social and legal reform to impact embedded hatred in our culture, and yet we still are exposed to public hate promoters on a daily basis.

Yes, it will take a village to stop weight discrimination.

Yes, it will take a social movement to end it.

Yes, it takes parents and teachers to educate the next generation.

And yes, you should no longer tolerate discrimination in any form.

The question becomes how to intervene when you are a target of obesity hatred? How do you make this kind of prejudice stop?

Most of these incidents occur spontaneously. All the preplanning in the world will not give you the perfect retort when you are dumbfounded by someone else's cruelty.

Often these incidents occur from strangers that you will likely never see again. Other times, these incidents occur in completely acceptable social contexts such as late night television, talk radio, party conversation.

Most often, they have not done anything illegal. Rude? Yes. Hurtful? Yes. Against the law? No. Where do you go to report a disapproving glare in a restaurant, an insult from a passing car, a person who changes direction rather than talk to you?

Maybe you can speak directly to a person making inappropriate remarks about your weight. It's a risk; the confrontation could make things worse. If it's safe, try and speak out or call for help when a child or disabled person is being ridiculed.

I could have said to the lady glaring at me in the restaurant, "Can I help you, I notice you are staring at me". It would have made her aware of her unsocial behavior. It would not have changed what she believed about obese people.

I would have been foolish to try to chase down a carload of strangers to confront them about yelling insults. I suppose I could have called the police if I had the presence of mind to get a license number, but I did not.

If you say or do nothing, these incidents begin to accumulate in your psyche and erode your self-esteem. Consciously, you feel horrible about yourself. Unconsciously, you may decide the abusers are correct.

We are here to experience emotion – good, bad and ugly. We are here to feel each moment with the full depths of our hearts, and minds and bodies. We are here to help each other, not to harm each other. We are here to heal and recover with each other's support.

We are here to be together. As one mass of connected, communicating, loving human energy.

Accept nothing less.

Obesity Comes Out Of The Closet

Follow these guiding principles if you have been discriminated against because of your weight:

Do not identify with the abuser, do not become like them, do not copy their behavior toward anyone else.

Reframe in your mind who they are, take away some of the importance you have given them.

The best way to feel better about yourself when you have experienced obesity-hatred is to "consider the source", as my mother used to say. Discredit them in your mind. Just because this is your boss, or your neighbor or a celebrity does not make them right. People who express unprovoked hatred towards others, who discriminate, who spew verbal garbage are troubled, disturbed people. They're not smart, they're just loud.

Speak up against weight discrimination. Tell people to stop. Say you won't tolerate this anymore. Tell them this is hatred and it makes THEM look ugly. Don't put yourself in danger, however. History has shown us many thousands and millions of hate crimes that ended with someone being physically maimed or murdered.

Go public. Tell what happened. Talk to your friends and family, your newspaper, the store owner, the Internet forum, your congressional representatives. Sometimes you may need an advocate or attorney. Most of the time, you need a friend.

Educate a child about what kindness is, and how you practice it on a daily basis.

Section Five

This Is What I Maybe Know For Sure

Chapter

20

This Is What I Maybe Know For Sure

"Namaste - The divine in me honors the divine in you"

You ask me if I'm "cured"? The answer is no, I am not, but I am better. What ailed me was not a disease, but a human condition. There are days when I am light, and bright and easy and days when I am dark and brooding and low. Sometimes I laugh, sometimes I cry. Most days I feel better when I move; some days I am sore and I rest. Overall, I have more really good days and fewer really bad days.

It's been a little over a year since that silent "pop" in my brain. I weigh 55 pounds less than I did at that moment, and 75 pounds less than at my heaviest weight. I still have 80 pounds to go to be lean and healthy and to get that drop-dead designer pantsuit I've always wanted. I have very little pain and take very little medication now. My goal is to take none. My energy is pretty good most days.

I have wrinkles in places that I didn't know wrinkled. Instead of miracle weight-loss ads, I now read miracle ads for non-surgical skin tightening. I don't believe them either, but if you want to send me some, I'll try it and report back to you.

I still overeat spontaneously. The other difficult day, I walked into the house, took out the gluten-free brownie mix, and methodically baked and ate two rows of brownies. I "needed" a brownie. It wasn't the best coping mechanism, but it worked, and it was, as we say in medicine, self-limited. The next day I ate normally without a second thought.

Some days I don't feel like walking, or meditating or socializing. I let it be.

Life has a balance now that it never had before.

I wish I could tell you that my struggle is over and that eating, and exercising and walking past chocolate chip cookies is easy.

I wish I could tell you that my knowledge is complete and I understand what was 'wrong' with me and with you and why we have fat bodies.

I wish I could tell you that the world will read this and understand that you, and I and all of us are human with souls, and wants, and emotions, and families and friends.

I wish I could tell you I have the "answer".

I can tell you that it is easier than ever before to manage my weight. I can identify an emotional eating pattern. I can forgive myself an extra treat and resume a nurturing, healthy way of living a moment later.

I have learned that I am not my body.

I am a divine being with an imperfect physical body.

I never thought I would go through the physical and emotional and spiritual changes I've been through. I don't feel old, or fat, or thin, or smart, or dumb, or silly or serious. I feel loved. I feel complete. I feel full.

When I look in the mirror, I am surprised. A middle-aged, gray-haired, overweight lady with kind eyes and a saggy neck looks back at me. There is calmness in her face. As if to say, we are one, you and I.

When I take her out walking on a beautiful day, the sky is bluer; the birds sing sweetly, the breeze comforts me. I could stay forever. There is no yesterday of pain. Only the now of beauty.

It is the same experience when I hear your story in my office.

Now you have heard mine.

The divine in me honors the divine in you and wishes you the same wholeness and satiety. We are one.

Resources

R esources are available online for all to see at
www.obesefromtheheart.com

There are many excellent resources for emotional, physical and spiritual healing for obese people available in print and video and on the internet; many more than can be listed here.

These are tools I use myself and suggest to my patients. There is a range of expenses – many of these are available in abbreviated form for free; many are downloadable. A few are very expensive, and are marked as such. There is no formula here other than experimentation. If you find something that works for you, go with it. Keep looking for the next resource that will help you and the next and the next. Remember, this is a process, not a procedure.

Overall Health and Nutrition:

- **Mark Hyman, M.D.**, www.drhyman.com is a leading expert on "Functional Medicine", a medical philosophy of disease prevention and healthy living. In The UltraMind Solution: Fix Your Broken Brain by Healing Your Body First, Dr. Hyman identifies the causes of many mood and memory symptoms, and suggests inexpensive and easily implemented changes. If you are extremely obese, start with minor changes and adjust to them slowly.

- **Andrew Weil, M.D.**, www.drweil.com is the father of alternative medicine for the masses. When I do not know what a supplement is, or which supplement to choose, this is the place. Good sound medical advice, comprehensive alternative treatments.

- **Sandra Cabot, M.D.**, www.liverdoctor.com has a wonderful program for obese persons with fatty liver disease and/or hepatitis. A very clear explanation about why your liver gets sick from your weight, which foods to eat and which ones to avoid, and what kinds of supplements will help.

- **David A. Kessler, M.D.**, former Chief of the Food and Drug Administration, discusses how the American food industry is contributing to the epidemic of obesity. The End of Overeating: Taking Control of the Insatiable American Appetite is a great book that helps you to understand the factors even if not all of them are under your direct control. www.theendofovereatingbook.com (plus he's got a chocolate chip cookie story too – must be the Tollhouse™ Generation!)

Emotions

- One of the best overall books for understanding how your emotions intertwine with your body and spirit is by psychiatrist Judith Orloff, M.D. I recommend that patients begin with *Positive Energy: 10 Extraordinary Prescriptions for Transforming Fatigue, Stress, and Fear Into Vibrance, Strength, and Love*. Her newest book, *Emotional Freedom: Liberate Yourself from Negative Emotions and Transform Your Life* addresses how to deal with parts of your life that drain your energy. www.judithorloff.com

The next two books can help you to see how much energy is used by different levels of emotion. Using these books, you can view emotional ladders from depression to joy, and step up, one step at a time. Normal is a range of emotions, not one single emotion all day long.

- **David R. Hawkins, M.D., Ph.D.** *Power vs Force: The Hidden Determinants of Human Behavior* 1995: Veritas Publishing.

- **Esther and Jerry Hicks.** *The Astonishing Power of Emotions: Let Your Feelings Be Your Guide.* I am more interested in the very great wisdom of material in this book than whether or not Esther Hicks is really channeling a consciousness from spirit. www.abraham-hicks.com

Anxiety And Panic

- **Belleruth Naparstek**, LISW www.healthjourneys.com The mother of guided imagery provides comprehensive audio programs and lots of free downloads. Listen to the audio any way you can – if you cannot set aside an hour of relaxation or if you are very stressed or anxious, listen in parts and pieces through the day – 10 minutes at a time, while getting dressed, working, etc. Try and get through the entire CD once a day – I have one lady who listens 15 min in the morning while getting dressed, 15 minutes at lunchtime, and 30 min at night after she gets into bed. She is relaxed at work, and no longer struggling with her supervisor, and tells me she's never yet heard the ending!

- **Master Chunyi Lin**, www.springforestqigong.com. When you feel overwhelmed with too much energy it generally means you have too much energy in your head. Try this technique: drop your shoulders, place your hands on your belly button and take long gentle deep breaths. Dropping your shoulders is very important - actually it's a trick. Remember to drop your shoulders. Good luck! When having an anxiety attack drink a glass of cold water, take long gentle deep breaths, step outside and get some fresh air and try not to focus on that emotion. Instead, feel how good you feel.

Depression

- If this is a crisis and you or someone you know is in danger, please call USA National Suicide Hotlines Toll-Free / 24 hours / 7 days a week
1-800-SUICIDE (1-800-784-2433);
1-800-273-TALK (1-800-273-8255);
TTY: 1-800-799-4TTY (4889)

- **James Gordon, M.D.**, former Chair of the National Institutes of Health Office on Alternative Medicine, www.jamesgordonmd. com has written a wonderful 7-step approach to dealing with depression called Unstuck: Your Guide to the Seven Stage Journey Out of Depression (Penguin Press).

- **Carol Tuttle** www.caroltuttle.com is a faith-based energy practitioner who has spectacular tapes on depression, anxiety, parenting and money woes. Her description of interrupting her negative thoughts while walking around in her kitchen is the best I've heard.

Connecting With Soul

- Israel 'IZ' Kamakawiwo'Ole 'Somewhere Over The Rainbow' on YouTube www.youtube.com/watch?v=0ltAGuuru7Q Thanks IZ!

- If you can only look at one resource, this is the one. Jill Bolte Taylor, Ph.D. A Stroke of Insight - www.drjilltaylor.com -This Harvard neuroanatomist discusses what happened when she had a nearly fatal stroke and lost her left brain function. Available in print or see the famous 18-minute video of her talk at the TED meeting www.TED.com

Creativity

- **www.playingforchange.com** Music producer Mark Johnson takes street musicians from all over the world and connects them in music, in spirit and in hope in this amazing documentary and set of videos.

- **Oriah Mountain Dreamer.** *What We Ache For: Creativity and the Unfolding of Your Soul* Harper San Francisco, 2005. www.oriahmountaindreamer.com

- **Mark David Gerson.** *The Voice of the Muse: Answering the Call to Write.* Santa Fe, NM: Light Lines Media, 2008. www.markdavidgerson.com

Energy Healing

Energy techniques include acupuncture, acupressure, reiki, EFT, Tai Chi, Qi Gong, and many others. Some practitioners are very experienced and well-trained. Spend time online researching the technique you are interested in, and talk to others who have experienced and benefitted from both the technique and the practitioner.

- **Emotional Freedom Technique** www.emofree.com Invented by Stanford engineer Gary Craig, an efficient, effective way to deliver full meridian acupressure tapping on yourself in times of distress. Impressive series of thousands of case reports. Can be learned online for free.

- **Donna Eden and David Feinstein** www.innersource.net are experts in the fields of energy medicine and energy psychology. Their training offers a comprehensive explanation to the meridians, but may be too detailed for some non-practitioners.

- **Healing Codes** – Invented by Alex Loyd, Ph.D, this is a focused energy technique that works on areas of the brain that contribute to distress and disease such as the hypothalamic-pituitary axis, frontal lobe regions, etc. Nice testimonial from co-owner Dr. Ben Johnson about how his Lou Gehrig's Disease remitted using these codes. They do work, but they are VERY EXPENSIVE and require diligence to do the codes three times daily for weeks to months, even though they are short. www.thehealingcodes.com

Energy, Exercise And Detoxification

Your body is designed to move. Even if you are hundreds of pounds overweight and unable to ambulate, you will find some movement here that you can do.

- **Walking** – start by walking 5-10 minutes at a time. As you build up tolerance, increase THE NUMBER OF TIMES A DAY, not distance. It is better to do three 10-minute walks a day then one 30-minute walk with sitting the rest of the day when you are very overweight.

- Master Chunyi Lin – Spring Forest Qi Gong - www.springforestqigong.com – The first QiGong DVD is for beginners and can be used by those who are extremely sedentary or ill, even bed or homebound or oxygen-dependent. You can begin in a chair or lying down.

- For DETOX, I recommend Francisco and Daisy Lee Garripoli's QiGong for Cleansing DVD. Once you learn this program, it is only 9 minutes and you can identify areas of illness that need additional work. www.wujiproductions.com/products/qigong-for-cleansing-dvd.htm

- www.bigyogaonline.com is the yoga of choice for obese persons. I love yoga, but every time I tried to do yoga, my stomach got in the way or I couldn't bend over. Check out the FAQ section for pictures of Meera demonstrating the Sun Salute.

Grief

Most Hospice and Palliative Medicine programs and many religious institutions have bereavement coordinators or groups – you can begin to work with a bereavement counselor before someone dies or years after. Professional grief counseling organizations on the internet will have lists of providers in your area.

- **Neale Donald Walsch** For people who believe in life after death, I recommend Home with God In a Life That Never Ends, part of the Conversations with God series. www.nealedonaldwalsch.com

- If you are a family survivor of someone who committed suicide, connect with a fantastic organization called Survivors of Suicide. There are groups and online support available. The reality of losing someone to suicide is that only people who have also gone through this will fully understand your experience. www.survivorsofsuicide.com

- **Pet Loss** – famed animal communicator Elizabeth Severino has a lovely book The Animals' Viewpoint on Dying, Death, and Euthanasia. www.beyond1.com

Illness

Illness requires medical care. Anyone who tells you otherwise puts you at risk. However, illness prevention and resolution of chronic illness requires identifying underlying physical issues and correcting them through lifestyle, medication and monitoring. The Institute for Functional Medicine represents a growing group of physicians and health-care providers who incorporate prevention and lifestyle into disease management. www.functionalmedicine.org

Life Purpose And Spiritual Healing

- **Dr. Wayne W. Dyer**, *Change Your Thoughts - Change Your Life: Living the Wisdom of the Tao.* There is more to life than being on a treadmill all day long trying to keep things under control. I love the CD's in my car – listening to them transforms my ride, and thus, transforms my day. Thank you Dr. Dyer! www.drwaynedyer. com

- **Gay Hendricks, Ph.D.**, revives a classic meaning-of-life exercise in his book *Five Wishes: How Answering One Simple Question Can Make Your Dreams Come True.* If you were on your deathbed, would you consider your life a success? And if not, why not? www.hendricks.com

- **Martha Beck Ph.D.**, *Finding Your Own North Star: Claiming the Life You Were Meant to Live.* If there were awards for common sense, this would be the winner. www.marthabeck.com

- **Louise Hay**, founder of Hay House Publishing, and driving force in mind-body-spirit psychology for years. In her book *You Can Heal Your Life*, Louise correlated illnesses with emotions. I always read the correlations aloud to patients with chronic illness to see if it rings true. Her affirmations are simply beautiful and always uplifting.

Meditation

Prayer is asking for help; meditation is listening for the answer

- An easy place to begin to learn about meditation is www. meditationsociety.com

- For people who have a hard time quieting their minds, assisted meditations are helpful. They incorporate sound, movement and video, and provide the benefits of relaxation and meditation. You don't have to work to quiet your mind; you can just put your headphones on. It works for me.

- www.mediheaven.com - computer guided audio and visual meditations that will transport you from 4 minutes to 30 minutes. Try "Rapid Relaxation" while at work, or during the day when you only have a few minutes.

- www.centerpointe.com - You can retrain your brain to stop the cycle of automatic thinking and worrying and overreacting by using this method. Holosync technology involves the same sound entering your ears at two different frequencies – something the brain finds very confusing. In order to make sense of the discrepancy, your brain actually grows new neurons in underused areas. I play it every night when I get into bed, and the next morning I am positively serene. Needs headphones. EXPENSIVE OVER TIME.

- PATHS Mind Energetics - A computer guided visual and audio meditation that uses binary code to suggest positive changes to your brain. Fun to watch and listen to. Honestly, I have no idea why it works, but I can tell you from both personal and patient experience that it absolutely does overcome resistance and allow healing. CAN BE EXPENSIVE TO BUY WITH ADDITIONAL MONTHLY SERVICE FEE. www.quantumpsychpaths.com - (DISCLOSURE - This is my personal page – 100% of the proceeds from sales of the PATHS program from this site will be donated to charity through the Quantum Psych Foundation chartered in 2009)

- EVOX by Zyto – Clearing Emotional Roadblocks Using Voice Repatterning. This is an amazing biofeedback type machine using voice recordings and lights to feedback and eliminate emotional blocks. It got me writing this book again! VERY EXPENSIVE to buy, look for a local practitioner. www.zyto.com/Products/Evox. aspx

Memory And Brain Health

The most frequent complaint I hear from obese patients is that they are losing their memory. Here are some steps you can take immediately to regain your normal brain function.

Begin by visiting Daniel Amen M.D.'s website www.amenclinics. com and view the pictures of SPECT scans of different brain conditions. A SPECT scan is an image of how your brain is functioning – areas that look like holes do not mean you are missing a chunk of brain – it means you have very little activity there, as if it's asleep.

Look at the normal brain – this is a healthy younger adult resting in the scanner. Blue activity is relaxed baseline. Higher activity levels are red. In the resting normal scan, a little bit of red activity may be associated with dreaming or daydreaming.

Now look at the Bipolar brain or the Attention Deficit Disorder brain – wild screaming amounts of red activity – which is exactly what people experience in their brain.

Once you understand what is going on in your brain, you will be better equipped to select supplements and regimens that will help you. Here are some brain treatments that are both effective and affordable:

Brain exercise has been shown to slow and even arrest certain types of age-related memory problems. They certainly improve menopause or disease-related brain fog.

- www.happy-neuron.com These folks will show you the areas of your brain where you are having problems and let you exercise them extra!

- Physical exercise is your single best defense against dementia. See the movement section.

- Brain anti-inflammatory: Here's the great news. A food supplement has been developed that appears to influence inflammation in the brain and may slow down progression of various dementias.

The active ingredient is a protein isolated from colostrum – the first breast milk that is rich in immune-helping proteins. The US version is Cognisure from Metagenix – side effects are minimal. About $50 per month, but how much would you pay to get your memory back? Works on brain fog too. (and seemed to help my husband's plantar fasciitis!). Look on the internet for a supplier near you.

- Two easily affordable and easily obtainable supplements for your brain health are Vitamin D3 (the "sunshine" vitamin) and 3-omega fatty acids (fish oil). Talk to your physician about having your D levels tested, particularly if you have depression or anxiety, live in a low sun climate, have renal disease, or are African-American.

- Regarding 3-omega fatty acids, look for the no mercury or PCB brands, and try the "no-burp" type if possible. Unless you live in Scandinavia and are eating sardines three times a day, you probably don't have high levels of 3-omega fatty acids. This is the "lube and oil" of your brain. 1000 mg twice daily if it's okay with your doctor.

Men

Dave Romanelli describes his book *Yeah Dave's Guide to Living in the Moment: Getting to Ecstasy through Wine, Chocolate and Your IPOD Playlist* as Deepak Chopra meets Cheech and Chong. It's a great guide for anyone, but men seem to really understand it. www.yeahdave.com

Pain

- Qi Gong: The Lotus Exercise for Self Healing - Acupuncturist Michael Costa has this You Tube video that will stimulate your energy and relax your pain in only 3 minutes. I recommend that you go through this 2-3 times in a row for maximum benefit. http://www.youtube.com/watch?v=rUsUrOaeM1c

- Tai Chi, Qigong, Reiki, EFT, acupuncture, acupressure, and massage are also excellent treatments for pain. Chronic pain requires chronic treatment. The benefit of these treatments is that your body does not become resistant to them, and the treatments continue to work, unlike painkiller medications. Frequency Specific Microcurrent is the gentlest of all current devices under the TENS classification. Works well for neuropathic pain such as shingles, fibromyalgia. May be difficult to find a practitioner in every area. www.frequencyspecific.com

Relaxation Techniques

There's no escaping this. Every book and magazine you read, every therapist you ask, every program you watch – everywhere you go, you will be told to work on relaxation. That's right WORK on relaxing. It takes planning and practice. It's your next best addiction.

- **Breathe.** When we are upset, we unconsciously hold our breaths or breathe extra-shallowly. Figures, doesn't it? Just when you need to slow down and take a deep breath, your anger/anxiety/ depression/stress has you doing the opposite.

- **Calming breaths** - Yoga breaths - inhale slowly through your nose and exhale slowly through your mouth. Do this at least 3 times.

- **Massaging breaths** - From Tai Chi or Qi Gong, squeeze your stomach/abdomen in at the end of an exhale and imagine your internal organs being massaged.

- **"Five Breaths" from Mark Hyman, M.D.**, The UltraMind Solution…5 deep breaths – inhale slowly to the count of 5, exhales slowly to the count of 5. Do this 5 times a day.

- **"Soft Belly"** from James Gordon, M.D., Unstuck….inhale slowly into your abdomen to the word "soft", exhale slowly and relax your abdomen to the word "belly". For as long as it takes to relax.

- **Connected breathing** – natural breathing has a "catch", or pause, between the inhale and the exhale. In connected breathing, you move yourself from inhale to exhale without that pause. Kind of like hyperventilating, except you are breathing slowly. Do this 20-100 breaths once daily. If you get dizzy or tingly, slow it down.

- **SING** – the best breathwork in the world – singing at the top of your lungs will increase your oxygen and your energy, and will increase your creativity too. Ok, I admit I have to keep the windows rolled up in the car or someone would call emergency ;-)

- **LAUGHTER** – Norman Cousins wrote about his own healing experience with laughter in Anatomy of an Illness, where he talked about his pain remitting after watching Marx Brothers movies. "I made the joyous discovery that ten minutes of genuine belly laughter had an anesthetic effect and would give me at least two hours of pain-free sleep".

- **EVERYTHING ELSE** - Massage, aromatherapy, reiki, relaxed walking, yoga, tai chi, stretching, meditation, prayer, reading, petting your animal, gardening, painting, listening to music, sex, a cuppa tea, sitting outside on a beautiful day….pick your relaxation, invent your own, share your pleasure with someone you love. Your brain chemicals will thank you.

Sex

Dr. Mia Rose has a terrific website that will help you learn about the physical, the emotional and the spiritual sides of sex. Don't be fooled by the name; there's a men's section also. www.better-sex-4-women.com

A lot about sex is in your mind – these will help you get in the mood. Sex takes concentration:

- Guided imagery and meditation tapes (www.mediheaven.com has a nice one)

- Tantric sex (see Mia's site – the ultimate mind over matter)

- Erotica

A lot about sex is in your body – start to work with your physical sensation using these:

- Yoga www.bigyogaonline.com

- Kegel exercises strengthen the pelvic floor and work equally well for men and women. The basic exercise involves squeezing pelvic muscles sufficient to cut off a flow of urine 200 times a day. Well, at least you won't be thinking about how depressed you are!

Two sites with good instructions:

- Women - www.childbirth.org/articles/kegel.html

- Men - http://socyberty.com/sexuality/kegel-exercises-for-men-to-improve-your-sexual-performance

Cushions – you may need support for a comfortable position during sex due to obesity or pain – these folks make great cushions

- www.liberator.com

Vibrators – patients with obesity, diabetes, back problems or medical illnesses may need more intense stimulation. There are a number of sites that sell sex toys and vibrators:

- This one is both reliable and discreet – although might seem a little shocking - www.freddyandeddy.com (not tied to the porn industry)

- Look for brands that specifically state they're phthalate-free, like Je Joue -http://jejoue.com

There are also approved medical devices available for men and women with sexual dysfunction that may require prescription such as www.eros-therapy.com . Most urologists and gynecologists are familiar with the available devices and their indications.

Trauma

For patients who have been traumatized, I recommend a combination of anxiety and depression treatments centered on stopping a cycle of repetitive thoughts. Reframing psychotherapy is crucial. Some patients will also need bereavement resources. Multiple treatment modalities are available, and should be discussed with your therapist or psychiatrist.

Any person who experiences an overwhelming trauma such as a hurricane, fire, car accident, or violent or war crime needs crisis counseling. You may also need crisis counseling if your loved one experienced the trauma. Most police and fire departments have local crisis counselors they can recommend, as does the Red Cross and other rescue organizations. Look online for specialized treatment groups.

- For victims of violent crime, contact NOVA, the National Organization for Victims Assistance 1-800-TRY-NOVA. Online at www.trynova.org

- For returning veterans, contact the National Center for Post-Traumatic Stress Disorder, run by the US Department of Veterans Affairs www.ptsd.va.gov . From their website: If you are in crisis, please go to your nearest Emergency Room, call 911, or call 1-800-273-TALK (1-800-273-8255) to talk to someone right now.

- For rape trauma, look for a local rape crisis center or contact the National Sexual Assault Hotline at 1.800.656.HOPE (4673). Online at http://centers.rainn.org

- For domestic violence, look for a local domestic violence center or contact the National Domestic Violence Hotline at 1.800.799. SAFE (7233) 1.800.787.3224 (TTY). Online at www.ndvh.org

I do not recommend or endorse any quick weight loss products including, but not limited to: diets, supplements, exercise programs, or medications.

None of them worked for me.

Go forth in good mental health!

CPSIA information can be obtained
at www.ICGtesting.com
Printed in the USA
BVHW081651081219
565990BV00002B/219/P

9 780982 524817